W9-AVW-052

Neonatal Encephalopathy and Cerebral Palsy

DEFINING THE PATHOGENESIS AND PATHOPHYSIOLOGY

The American College of
Obstetricians and Gynecologists

Women's Health Care Physicians

American Academy
of Pediatrics

DEDICATED TO THE HEALTH OF ALL CHILDREN™

Neonatal Encephalopathy and Cerebral Palsy: Defining the Pathogenesis and Pathophysiology was developed under the direction of the Task Force on Neonatal Encephalopathy and Cerebral Palsy. The information in *Neonatal Encephalopathy and Cerebral Palsy: Defining the Pathogenesis and Pathophysiology* should not be viewed as a body of rigid rules. The guidelines are general and intended to be adapted to many different situations, taking into account the needs and resources particular to the locality, the institution, or the type of practice. Variations and innovations that improve the quality of patient care are to be encouraged rather than restricted. The purpose of these guidelines will be well served if they provide a firm basis on which local norms may be built.

Studies were reviewed and evaluated for quality according to the method outlined by the U.S. Preventive Services Task Force:

I Evidence obtained from at least one properly designed randomized controlled trial.

II-1 Evidence obtained from well-designed controlled trials without randomization.

II-2 Evidence obtained from well-designed cohort or case–control analytic studies, preferably from more than one center or research group.

II-3 Evidence obtained from multiple time series with or without the intervention. Dramatic results in uncontrolled experiments also could be regarded as this type of evidence.

III Opinions of respected authorities, based on clinical experience, descriptive studies, or reports of expert committees.

Library of Congress Cataloging-in-Publication Data
Neonatal encephalopathy and cerebral palsy : defining the pathogenesis & pathophysiology : a report / by the American College of Obstetricians and Gynecologists' Task Force on Neonatal Encephalopathy and Cerebral Palsy and the American College of Obstetricians and Gynecologists and the American Academy of Pediatrics.
 p. ; cm.
Includes bibliographical references and index.
 ISBN 0-915473-91-7
 1. Cerebral palsied children. 2. Brain-damaged children. 3. Infants (Newborn)—Diseases.
 [DNLM: 1. Cerebral Palsy—etiology—Infant, Newborn. 2. Brain Damage, Chronic—etiology—Infant, Newborn. 3. Cerebral Palsy—diagnosis—Infant, Newborn. 4. Cerebral Palsy—physiopathology—Infant, Newborn. 5. Prenatal Diagnosis. WS 342 N438 2002] I. American College of Obstetricians and Gynecologists. Task Force on Neonatal Encephalopathy and Cerebral Palsy. II. American Academy of Pediatrics.

RJ496.C4 N44 2002
618.92'836—dc21

2002015572

Copyright © January 2003 by the American College of Obstetricians and Gynecologists, 409 12th Street, SW, PO Box 96920, Washington, DC 20090-6920. All rights reserved. No part of this publication may be reproduced, stored in a retrieval system, or transmitted, in any form or by any means, electronic, mechanical, photocopying, recording, or otherwise, without prior written permission from the publisher.

Copies of *Neonatal Encephalopathy and Cerebral Palsy: Defining the Pathogenesis and Pathophysiology* can be ordered through the ACOG Distribution Center by calling toll free 800-762-2264. Orders also can be placed from the ACOG web site at www.acog.org or sales.acog.org.

12345/76543

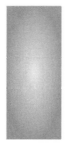

CONTENTS

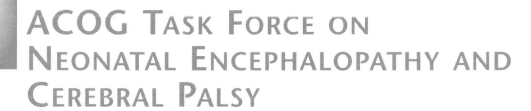

ACOG Task Force on Neonatal Encephalopathy and Cerebral Palsy

Gary D.V. Hankins, MD, FACOG, Chair
Maternal–Fetal Medicine
University of Texas Medical Branch
Galveston, Texas

Mary D'Alton, MD, FACOG
Maternal–Fetal Medicine
Director of Obstetrics and Gynecology
Columbia Presbyterian Medical Center
New York, New York

Richard Depp, III, MD, FACOG
Maternal–Fetal Medicine
Dept. of Obstetrics and Gynecology
MCP–Hahnemann of Drexel University
Philadelphia, Pennsylvania

Mark Ira Evans, MD, FACOG
Medical Genetics
Dept. of Obstetrics and Gynecology
MCP–Hahnemann of Drexel University
Philadelphia, Pennsylvania

Roger K. Freeman, MD, FACOG
Maternal–Fetal Medicine
Long Beach, California

Larry Gilstrap, MD, FACOG
Maternal–Fetal Medicine
Dept. of Obstetrics and Gynecology
University of Texas
Houston, Texas

Richard P. Green, MD, FACOG
Obstetrics and Gynecology
Washington, DC

James A. McGregor, MD, FACOG
Maternal–Fetal Medicine
Tucson, Arizona

Karin B. Nelson, MD
Child Neurology
Chief, Neuroepidemiology Branch
National Institute of Neurological Disorders and Stroke
National Institute of Health
Bethesda, Maryland

Susan Ramin, MD, FACOG
Maternal–Fetal Medicine
Dept. of Obstetrics and Gynecology
University of Texas
Houston, Texas

Robert Resnik, MD, FACOG
Maternal–Fetal Medicine
University of California
San Diego School of Medicine
La Jolla, California

Louis Weinstein, MD, FACOG
Maternal–Fetal Medicine
Dept. of Obstetrics and Gynecology
Medical College of Ohio
Toledo, Ohio

Ex Officio Member

Frank C. Miller, MD, FACOG
Maternal–Fetal Medicine
Dept. of Obstetrics and Gynecology
University of Kentucky College of Medicine
Lexington, Kentucky

AAP Liaison Members

James Lemons, MD, FAAP
Director, Section of Neonatal–Perinatal Medicine
Department of Pediatrics
Indiana University School of Medicine
Indianapolis, Indiana

Michael E. Speer, MD, FAAP
Professor of Pediatrics
Division of Neonatology
Baylor College of Medicine
Houston, Texas

ACOG STAFF

Stanley Zinberg, MD, MS, FACOG
Debra Hawks, MPH
Rebecca Carlson, MS
Meriam Sellers-Haynes

ACOG TASK FORCE CONSULTANTS

A. James Barkovich, MD
Professor of Radiology, Neurology, Pediatrics and Neurosurgery
University of California, San Francisco School of Medicine
San Francisco, California

Kurt Benirschke, MD
Professor Emeritus of Pathology and Reproductive Medicine
University of California, San Diego Medical Center
San Diego, California

Robert R. Clancy, MD
Pediatric Regional Epilepsy Program
The Children's Hospital of Pennsylvania
Philadelphia, Pennsylvania

Gabrielle A. deVeber, MD
Director, Perinatal Stroke Pediatric Ischemic Stroke Registry
Toronto, Ontario, Canada

Ronald Gibbs, MD
Maternal–Fetal Medicine
Department of Obstetrics and Gynecology
University of Colorado Health Sciences Center
Denver, Colorado

Marjorie R. Grafe, MD
Professor, Department of Pathology
University of Texas Medical Branch
Galveston, Texas

Gregory J. Locksmith, MD
Maternal–Fetal Medicine
Department of Obstetrics and Gynecology
University of Texas Medical Branch
Galveston, Texas

Jeffrey M. Perlman, MD, ChB
Professor of Pediatrics and Obstetrics and Gynecology
University of Texas Southwestern Medical Center at Dallas
Dallas, Texas

Julian N. Robinson, MD
Division of Maternal Fetal Medicine
New York Presbyterian Hospital
Columbia University
New York, New York

Dwight J. Rouse, MD
Maternal–Fetal Medicine
Division of Maternal–Fetal Medicine, Department of Obstetrics and
Gynecology, University of Alabama at Birmingham
Birmingham, Alabama

George R. Saade, MD
Maternal–Fetal Medicine
Professor, Department of Obstetrics and Gynecology
The University of Texas Medical Branch
Galveston, Texas

Diana E. Schendel, PhD
National Center on Birth Defects and Developmental Disabilities
Centers for Disease Control and Prevention
Atlanta, Georgia

Rodney E. Willoughby, Jr, MD
Pediatrics, Johns Hopkins University Hospital
Baltimore, Maryland

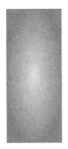

ENDORSEMENTS

The following federal agencies and professional organizations have reviewed, endorsed, and support this report:

- Centers for Disease Control and Prevention, U.S. Department of Health and Human Services
- Child Neurology Society (recommends as a valuable educational tool for its members)
- March of Dimes Birth Defects Foundation
- National Institute of Child Health and Human Development, National Institutes of Health, U.S. Department of Health and Human Services
- The Royal Australian and New Zealand College of Obstetricians and Gynaecologists
- Society for Maternal–Fetal Medicine
- Society of Obstetricians and Gynaecologists of Canada

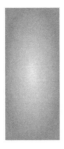

FOREWORD

Rapid advances in epidemiologic, maternal–fetal, and pediatric research have led to a revolution in thought and understanding about the causation of neonatal encephalopathy and cerebral palsy. Until recently, four nonspecific clinical signs, 1) meconium stained liquor, 2) nonreassuring fetal heart rate patterns, 3) low Apgar scores, and 4) neonatal encephalopathy, were often assumed to be adequate evidence of *birth asphyxia* and *hypoxic–ischemic* neonatal encephalopathy in the absence of objective criteria to show that a de novo acute hypoxic event had actually occurred during labor and delivery. In reality, these nonspecific peripartum signs, which first alert medical staff and parents to possible infant compromise, often are the sequelae of pathological processes established before labor.

New data, discussed in this report, confirm that intrapartum hypoxia is uncommonly the sole cause of neonatal encephalopathy or cerebral palsy. Less than a quarter of infants with neonatal encephalopathy have evidence of hypoxia or ischemia at birth and, therefore, it is inappropriate to label most newborns with encephalopathy as having hypoxic–ischemic neonatal encephalopathy. Similarly, the potential for misclassification of an infant with birth asphyxia is very great when the four nonspecific signs mentioned previously provide the main evidence for the diagnosis. These signs can follow both chronic hypoxic and nonhypoxic fetal pathology or may be associated with a normal long-term outcome. Although past studies have used these relatively weak clinical signs to diagnose acute hypoxia at birth, the validity of their conclusions may have been compromised when assessing long-term outcome after acute hypoxia or when attempts have been made to correlate neuroimaging patterns, many years after birth, with a presumed asphyxial event at the time of delivery. In the future, it will be necessary to either objectively clarify the likely cause and timing of any antenatal, intrapartum, neonatal, or pediatric neuropathology before the risks of adverse sequelae can be predicted or prove that the use of brain-imaging years after the event is a valid way to retrospectively diagnose the cause and timing of cerebral palsy.

The American College of Obstetricians and Gynecologists (ACOG) Task Force on Neonatal Encephalopathy has clearly delineated objective criteria to use when defining an acute intrapartum hypoxic event. These criteria should be examined before a label of birth asphyxia or hypoxic–ischemic encephalopathy is written into the infant's case notes and given to the parents as a diagnosis. Accurately defining the relatively uncommon event of intrapartum asphyxia, with its uncommon sequelae of neonatal encephalopathy and cerebral palsy, will allow for better definitions of the possible nonhypoxic causes of encephalopathy and cerebral palsy. Criticism of the management of labor should not be confused with cerebral palsy causation because the two often may not be linked.

The nine criteria endorsed by the ACOG Task Force in Chapter 8 emphasize that analysis of peripartum blood gases is essential to prove that hypoxia was present around birth. For a causative link to be established, a severe metabolic acidosis must occur in sequence with early neonatal encephalopathy and a type of cerebral palsy that could have been caused by hypoxia. Because intrapartum compromise can be simply a reflection of antenatal fetal pathology, known etiologies or strong associations with subsequent cerebral palsy should help to exclude primary intrapartum hypoxia as the likely cause. However, in seeking evidence for this fourth criterion, it should be remembered that most antenatal causes of cerebral palsy are currently undetectable during routine antenatal care and especially in retrospect. The five final criteria help to distinguish whether the intrapartum hypoxia, if present, is acute or chronic. Although individually nonspecific, most or all of these five signs will be present as a group in severe cases of acute intrapartum hypoxia.

These criteria have been refined from previous criteria recommended by ACOG and by a separate International Cerebral Palsy Task Force that published its consensus statement in the British Medical Journal in 1999.* The 1999 and 2003 Task Force reports are complementary and are not, except in occasional minor detail, in conflict. As Chairman of the 1999 consensus statement, I am delighted to see it updated and extended. Just as this current report is clearly stated to be a work in progress, the members of the 1999 Task Force hoped that other researchers would update the knowledge in this rapidly evolving area. Although the ACOG Task Force membership and consultant list contains many renowned names in maternal–fetal medicine, it also includes distinguished pediatricians, neuroepidemiologists, radiologists, and pathologists. This multidisciplinary approach is essential when examining the complex issues surrounding the many causes of neonatal encephalopathy and cerebral palsy.

I commend the altruism of the ACOG Task Force members who have spent many hundreds of hours, over 2 years, formulating this important and insightful report. The ACOG Task Force has met its goals admirably, displaying obvious care and effort. The ACOG/AAP report is the current state-of-the-art and is thoroughly referenced and evidence based. It is a scientifically detailed document that will give a better clinical understanding of the antecedents of neonatal encephalopathy and cerebral palsy to those who work in this field and to those who care for infants and children with these disabilities. By helping to define and understand causation of neonatal encephalopathy and cerebral palsy, this document may lead to clinical interventions that will reduce the rates of these serious pathologies. I warmly congratulate the members of the ACOG Task Force for a difficult task well done.

Alastair MacLennan, MD, FRCOG, FRANZCOG
Chair, International Cerebral Palsy Task Force
Professor, Obstetrics and Gynaecology
Adelaide University, Australia

*MacLennan A. A template for defining a casual relation between acute intrapartum events and cerebral palsy: international consensus statement. BMJ 1999;319:1054–9.

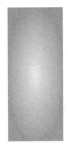

PREFACE

Advances in both science and technology, ranging from imaging modalities to advanced molecular biology techniques, indicate that most cases of neonatal encephalopathy and cerebral palsy do not originate during the process of labor and delivery. It is now accepted that most neonatal encephalopathy and cerebral palsy have their origins in developmental abnormalities, metabolic abnormalities, autoimmune and coagulation defects, infection, trauma, or combinations of these factors. The best evidence from multiple clinical epidemiologic studies confirms the overwhelming majority of cases of cerebral palsy do not result from isolated intrapartum hypoxia with resultant asphyxia and organ damage. In 2000, Dr. Frank Miller, then president of the American College of Obstetricians and Gynecologists (ACOG), initiated the Task Force on Neonatal Encephalopathy and Cerebral Palsy to address current evidence on the causes of neonatal encephalopathy. At that time Dr. Miller issued the following mission statement:

> "To create a multidisciplinary task force to review and consider the current state of scientific knowledge about the mechanisms and timing of possible etiologic events which may result in neonatal encephalopathy. The purpose of such review will be to produce a consensus statement, report or monograph for Fellows of the College which will succinctly summarize the neuroscience of neonatal encephalopathy and provide a framework for explaining to patients and the general public, in understandable language, medicine's ability and capacity (and limitations) to detect, treat or in any way affect the pathophysiologic mechanisms which result in neonatal encephalopathy."

Methods

The ACOG Task Force on Neonatal Encephalopathy and Cerebral Palsy was convened in 2000 and comprised several physicians with expertise in the various issues in this field. Liaison members from the American Academy of Pediatrics also were appointed. Beginning in 2000, the Task Force met four times over the span of 2 years. At the first meeting, members outlined the subject matter to be covered, identified clinicians and scientists with particular expertise in the field, and solicited written contributions based on an extensive review of the literature from those clinicians and scientists. At subsequent meetings, the Task Force evaluated the written material, reached consensus, recruited expert authors to write the sections, and reviewed all draft documents. Throughout the process, primary source documents were cited to the fullest extent possible.

Once the draft was completed, numerous federal agencies and professional organizations endorsed the report and have indicated support of the Task Force's review of the evidence and its recommendations as follows: Centers for Disease Control and Prevention, U.S. Department of Health and Human Services; the Child Neurology Society; March of Dimes Birth Defects Foundation; National Institute of Child Health and Human Development, National Institutes of Health, U.S. Department of Health and Human Services; The Royal Australian and New Zealand College of Obstetricians and Gynecologists; Society for Maternal–Fetal Medicine; and the Society of Obstetricians and Gynaecologists of Canada. The American Academy of Pediatrics continued to be involved throughout the project as a liaison and is a co-author of the report.

Task Force Goals

The Task Force identified four specific goals of overriding importance:

1. To broaden the understanding of neonatal encephalopathy, especially that which is associated with subsequent cerebral palsy, by summarizing the topic using the best available primary source scientific data and the expertise of highly qualified individuals who have been major contributors in the field

2. To develop recommendations for evaluation of the newborn with encephalopathy to assist the clinician in defining both the cause and timing of the encephalopathy

3. To identify areas in which further research is needed

4. To raise awareness of the need for standardization of terminology and precision in its use, which is imperative to allow meaningful research on neonatal encephalopathy and cerebral palsy

The Role of Intervention

The pathogenesis of cerebral palsy is complex and incompletely understood, making prevention—while desirable—elusive. Although the sensitivity and specificity of tests to identify variables associated with cerebral palsy are unrelated to the prevalence of cerebral palsy, both the positive and negative predictive values of tests used as markers of events—such as intrapartum hypoxia as a causal antecedent of cerebral palsy—are highly affected by disease prevalence. Accordingly, because cerebral palsy is a rare event, caution is urged in ascribing specific interventions designed to prevent its occurrence without a thorough cost–benefit analysis for both the pregnant woman, the fetus, and the woman's potential future pregnancies.

About This Document

The Task Force acknowledges that this publication is a work in progress; it incorporates advanced concepts as they are currently understood, and it serves as another building block toward our complete understanding of these important conditions and their predecessors. This document includes data from several epidemiologic studies that identify specific preconceptional, antepartum, intrapartum, and neonatal associations with both neonatal encephalopathy and with cerebral palsy. Interpreting and understanding these studies requires familiarity with terms such as relative risk, adjusted relative risk, sensitivity, specificity, positive predictive value, and negative predictive value. These and other terms used throughout the document are defined in the glossary.

Gary D. V. Hankins, MD, FACOG
Chair, Task Force on Neonatal Encephalopathy and Cerebral Palsy

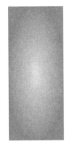

EXECUTIVE SUMMARY

The American College of Obstetricians and Gynecologists (ACOG) convened a Task Force on Neonatal Encephalopathy and Cerebral Palsy to collate and review the best scientific data available on the topic and to publish these findings. The American Academy of Pediatrics collaborated with ACOG on the Task Force and is a co-author of the final report. This executive summary covers important information and is intended to complement, not substitute, the full report.

Neonatal encephalopathy and its subset of hypoxic–ischemic encephalopathy (HIE) are conditions defined in and described for term and near-term infants. Neonatal encephalopathy is defined clinically on the basis of a constellation of findings to include a combination of abnormal consciousness, tone and reflexes, feeding, respiration, or seizures and can result from myriad conditions. Neonatal encephalopathy may or may not result in permanent neurologic impairment. It can be stated with certainty, however, that the pathway from an intrapartum hypoxic–ischemic injury to subsequent cerebral palsy must progress through neonatal encephalopathy.

In contrast, cerebral palsy is a chronic disability of central nervous system origin characterized by aberrant control of movement and posture, appearing early in life and not as a result of progressive neurologic disease. Research supports that spastic quadriplegia, especially with an associated movement disorder, is the only type of cerebral palsy associated with an acute interruption of blood supply. Purely dyskinetic or ataxic cerebral palsy, especially where there is an associated learning difficulty, commonly has a genetic origin and is not caused by intrapartum or peripartum asphyxia. Similarly, absent cerebral palsy, neither epilepsy, mental retardation, nor attention-deficit hyperactivity disorder are caused by birth asphyxia.

Historically, the factors used to define perinatal asphyxia, such as meconium-stained amniotic fluid and Apgar scores, were not specific to the disease process leading to neurologic damage. For instance, Nelson and associates have shown that use of nonreassuring fetal heart rate patterns to predict subsequent cerebral palsy had a 99% false-positive rate. Use of such nonspecific markers for perinatal asphyxia identifies a large number of individuals as being exposed to inappropriately diagnosed "perinatal asphyxia." Thus, it is not surprising that removing exposure to such nonspecific markers has failed to change the risk for the disease.

Epidemiologic studies have shown that only 19% of cases of neonatal encephalopathy met what were very nonstringent criteria for intrapartum hypoxia, with another 10% experiencing a significant intrapartum event that may have been associated with intrapartum hypoxia. Even with such inexact markers for intrapartum fetal hypoxia, they demonstrated that of all cases of neonatal encephalopathy, 69% had only antepartum risk factors, 25% had both antepartum and intrapartum risk factors, 4% had evidence of only intrapartum hypoxia without identified preconceptional or antepartum factors that might have contributed to neonatal encephalopathy, and 2% had no identified risk factors. Thus, approximately 70% of neonatal encephalopathy is secondary to events arising before the onset of labor. The overall incidence of neonatal encephalopathy attributable to intrapartum hypoxia, in the absence of any other preconceptional or antepartum abnormalities, is estimated to be approximately 1.6 per 10,000. It is again emphasized that HIE is but one subset of neonatal encephalopathy; other subsets include those resulting from prenatal stroke, infection, cerebral malformation, genetic disorders, and many other conditions.

The criteria to define an acute intrapartum event sufficient to cause cerebral palsy, as modified by this Task Force from the template provided by the International Cerebral Palsy Task Force, are listed as follows:*

Essential criteria (must meet all four)

1. Evidence of a metabolic acidosis in fetal umbilical cord arterial blood obtained at delivery (pH <7 and base deficit ≥12 mmol/L)

2. Early onset of severe or moderate neonatal encephalopathy in infants born at 34 or more weeks of gestation

3. Cerebral palsy of the spastic quadriplegic or dyskinetic type†

4. Exclusion of other identifiable etiologies such as trauma, coagulation disorders, infectious conditions, or genetic disorders

Criteria that collectively suggest an intrapartum timing (within close proximity to labor and delivery, eg, 0–48 hours) but are nonspecific to asphyxial insults

1. A sentinel (signal) hypoxic event occurring immediately before or during labor

2. A sudden and sustained fetal bradycardia or the absence of fetal heart rate variability in the presence of persistent, late, or variable decelerations, usually after a hypoxic sentinel event when the pattern was previously normal

3. Apgar scores of 0–3 beyond 5 minutes

4. Onset of multisystem involvement within 72 hours of birth

5. Early imaging study showing evidence of acute nonfocal cerebral abnormality

---

*Modified from MacLennan A. A template for defining a casual relation between acute intrapartum events and cerebral palsy: international consensus statement. BMJ 1999;319:1054–9.
†Spastic quadriplegia and, less commonly, dyskinetic cerebral palsy are the only types of cerebral palsy associated with acute hypoxic intrapartum events. Spastic quadriplegia is not specific to intrapartum hypoxia. Hemiparetic cerebral palsy, hemiplegic cerebral palsy, spastic diplegia, and ataxia are unlikely to result from acute intrapartum hypoxia (Nelson KB, Grether JK. Potentially asphyxiating conditions and spastic cerebral palsy in infants of normal birth weight. Am J Obstet Gynecol 1998;179:507–13.).

The Task Force recognizes that this summary will require updating as the scientific database and knowledge on this topic expands. Only with more complete understanding of the precise origins and pathophysiology of neonatal encephalopathy and cerebral palsy can logical hypotheses be designed and tested to reduce their occurrence. As such, we recommend several important areas of research that are detailed in the text of the full document. We encourage those engaged in research to pursue these areas, and others to exert influence to the degree possible to propel this to a high priority for funding and study.

Finally, we acknowledge our many consultants and support staff who made this project possible. Additionally, the input from and endorsement by the Centers for Disease Control and Prevention, U.S. Department of Health and Human Services; March of Dimes Birth Defects Foundation; National Institute of Child Health and Human Development, National Institutes of Health, U.S. Department of Health and Human Services; the Royal Australian and New Zealand College of Obstetricians and Gynaecologists; the Society for Maternal–Fetal Medicine; and the Society of Obstetricians and Gynaecologists of Canada has resulted in one of the most highly peer-reviewed and scientifically rigorous documents ever published on this topic.

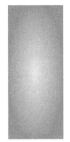

CHAPTER 1

BACKGROUND

Neonatal Encephalopathy and Cerebral Palsy: How They Differ in Major Gestational Age or Birth Weight Groups

Neonatal encephalopathy and hypoxic–ischemic encephalopathy (HIE) are conditions defined in and described for term (>37 completed weeks of gestation) and near-term (>34 completed weeks of gestation) infants. Most current evidence relating neonatal clinical neurologic findings to long-term risk is specific to term and near-term infants. Neurologic signs are more clearly recognizable and classifiable in mature newborn infants than in those born long before term. Most current evidence relating neonatal clinical neurologic findings to long-term risk is specific to term and near-term infants. The stages of development of various organ systems, including brain and immune systems, and the vulnerabilities of elements of these to injury range widely over the second half of gestation; the relative homogeneity of functional maturation in infants born at or near term permits clearer identification of biologic mechanisms. Finally, term and near-term infants constitute the majority of all births. Although term and near-term infants are at relatively low risk for cerebral palsy compared with very preterm infants, they still make up at least one half of all cases of cerebral palsy—and a much higher proportion of most other forms of long-term neurologic morbidity.

Infants of very low gestational age or birth weight are a tiny proportion of the birth population, but as a group they experience higher morbidity and mortality than more mature infants. Individually they are at high risk for cerebral palsy, and while a minority, constitute a disproportionate share of cases. Infants weighing less than 1,500 g at birth account for approximately one quarter of the cases of cerebral palsy. Very preterm babies have a variety of other neurologic, sensory, and behavioral disorders in addition to their high risk for motor disorders. Although they are more difficult to study in many regards and do not experience a defined clinical syndrome of neonatal encephalopathy, very preterm infants are obviously an extremely important group.

This document focuses on neonatal encephalopathy and HIE and later outcome in term and near-term infants. When evidence exists relating to very preterm infants, that information is provided in separate subsections.

Neonatal Encephalopathy: Epidemiology and Long-Term Neurologic Outcomes

Definition

Historically, assumptions about the role of adverse intrapartum events on the status of the newborn and neonate gave rise to the term hypoxic–ischemic encephalopathy to categorize a clinical syndrome observed primarily in infants born at term. These early definitions for HIE (postasphyxial encephalopathy, birth asphyxia, and perinatal asphyxia) described an array of abnormal neurologic findings evident within the first week of life in term infants believed to have experienced asphyxia during labor and delivery (1–5). The abnormal neonatal neurologic findings were fairly consistent and typically included clinical signs of abnormal states of consciousness, tone and reflexes, and respiratory function graded by severity of signs and symptoms, with the most severe state characterized by severe hypotonia, apnea, coma, and seizures.

Defining the presumed attributable exposure—intrapartum asphyxia—was much more problematic because often there were no direct measures of the primary insult (eg, cord compression, placental insufficiency, or abnormal uterine contractions), nor were many sensitive measures of its biochemical and neurologic sequelae routinely available—which remains true today (6–9). Thus, the criteria for exposure depended on secondary clinical signs and varied among studies—ranging from any one or an assortment of the following: birth asphyxia as recorded in the medical record, clinical markers of nonreassuring fetal status (eg, meconium in amniotic fluid or abnormal fetal heart rate during labor), laboratory markers of fetal acidosis (eg, umbilical cord blood pH or base excess), or markers of newborn status (eg, Apgar scores, time to spontaneous respiration, or time on assisted ventilation). These different criteria actually combined markers of an insult itself (eg, obstetric complications) with markers of a fetal–neonatal response to insult (eg, meconium or abnormal fetal heart rate) and markers of newborn neurologic status (eg, Apgar score)

(10). No data exist to support either the equivalence of these different criteria in terms of exposure to intrapartum asphyxia or whether they were actually specific to intrapartum asphyxia. Using any combination of these observable but nonspecific clinical signs as the criteria for asphyxia is not valid and may be misleading (10), creating enormous potential for misclassifying an infant as having sustained intrapartum asphyxia.

Appreciation for this potential source of error began to grow after reports demonstrated that many of these presumed markers for intrapartum asphyxia—specifically fetal acidemia (cord blood pH <7) (11–13); 1- and 5-minute Apgar scores (14, 15); abnormal fetal heart rate patterns in labor (16, 17); and meconium in the amniotic fluid (18, 19)—were poorly associated with adverse neurologic outcome. Of the conditions listed, possibly the best single marker for poor long-term neurologic outcome was a persistently low Apgar score (≤3) beyond 5 minutes and especially at 20 minutes (20). Nevertheless, these reports generally revealed that although some proportion of individuals who had these exposures had poor neurologic outcome, most had no short- or long-term neurologic dysfunction (ie, the markers showed low positive predictive value). In addition, most individuals who were neurologically abnormal were not exposed to these markers (ie, the markers showed low sensitivity). Thus, considered individually, these markers of exposure were neither sensitive nor reliable predictors of adverse neurologic outcome. It is clear, however, that neurologic damage, such as isolated mental retardation, attention deficit disorder, or seizure disorder, cannot be attributed to birth asphyxia in the absence of newborn encephalopathy. Further, cerebral palsy cannot be attributed to intrapartum events in the absence of newborn encephalopathy (21–27).

Substantial attention has been focused on asphyxial events as contributors to long-term neurologic deficit. An alternative perspective that focuses only on the neonatal neurologic symptoms has been advocated, identifying neonatal encephalopathy as a clinically defined syndrome of disturbed neurologic function in the earliest days of life in the term infant, manifested by difficulty initiating and maintaining respiration, depression of tone and reflexes, subnormal level of consciousness, and, often, seizures (21). This alternative perspective is extremely important for epidemiologic purposes because it both permits identification of affected infants on the basis of clinically observable data and imposes no assumptions about etiology of the disorder (22). Consequently, because there is no biased preselection of infants based on a presumed exposure, the true burden of neonatal encephalopathy in the population can be estimated, the full array of possible etiologic factors leading to neonatal encephalopathy (of which asphyxial events leading to HIE are a subset) can be investigated, and the full contribution of neonatal encephalopathy to long-term neurologic dysfunction can be assessed.

Incidence

The reported incidence of an array of conditions variously labeled birth asphyxia, HIE, or post-asphyxial encephalopathy in term or near-term infants ranges from 1 to 8 per 1,000 births. Investigators have reported an incidence rate for severe birth asphyxia (5-minute Apgar score ≤3) of 2.9 per 1,000 term infants (28) and for more moderate birth asphyxia (defined as a 5-minute Apgar score <7 because there were no other objective markers available) an incidence rate of 6.9 per 1,000 term infants (29). On the basis of a highly selected sample intended to exclude infants with neonatal neurologic disturbance presumably not related to asphyxia, another study reported an incidence rate for postasphyxial encephalopathy of 6 per 1,000 term infants (3). Other investigators reported incidence rates for HIE of 7.7 per 1,000 (from 1976 to 1980) and 4.6 per 1,000 (from 1984 to 1988), although the defining criteria for HIE comprised only clinical neurologic symptoms and did not include additional markers for some sort of asphyxial exposure (ie, closely approximating the definition for neonatal encephalopathy) (30). In comparison, on the basis of 41,000 births between 1959 and 1966 documented by the National Collaborative Perinatal Project, other investigators found a rate of 5.4 per 1,000 births for infants weighing more than 2,500 g and with adverse

neonatal signs similar to signs of neonatal encephalopathy (specifically, decreased activity after the first day of life, need for incubator care for 3 or more days, feeding problems, poor sucking ability, respiratory difficulty, or neonatal seizures) (31).

Because studies have used different criteria for defining neonatal encephalopathy (22), or its subset HIE, it is doubtful the resulting samples of subjects are equivalent (in terms of the etiology of their illness or neonatal clinical course, although they may overlap) or the reported rates are comparable. Additionally, given the broad range of birth years among the studies, these data may not reflect current clinical practice trends (more recent studies tend to report lower rates), but the differences in study designs make it impossible to judge. However, these data may demonstrate the effects on incidence rates of the degree of inclusiveness or exclusiveness among criteria for defining neonatal encephalopathy, with lower rates typically reported from studies in which the criteria were more exclusive. Perhaps the best recent estimates of the incidence of neonatal encephalopathy come from large, population-based studies that used restrictive (exclusive) criteria to define HIE and broad (inclusive) criteria to define neonatal encephalopathy. A review of three studies yielded a range of 1.9–3.8 per 1,000 for the combined diagnoses of HIE and neonatal encephalopathy, HIE representing a subset of neonatal encephalopathy (22). The best available evidence suggests an incidence rate for pure HIE (ie, neonatal encephalopathy with intrapartum hypoxia in the absence of any other preconceptional or antepartum abnormalities) of approximately 1.6 per 10,000 births (24).

Risk Factors

Historically, the incorrect assumptions that virtually all cases of neonatal encephalopathy resulted from intrapartum asphyxia impeded the search for other causes for neonatal encephalopathy, especially causes arising before the onset of labor. As already discussed, these assumptions often narrowly dictated the selection criteria for subjects (eg, only infants presumed to be exposed to intrapartum asphyxia), thus creating small, select samples not representative of all infants affected by neonatal encephalopathy. Typically, the studies also did not include a group of unaffected infants for comparison, so it was impossible to determine whether the perinatal characteristics of the study infants (if such data were even reported) differed in any way from a comparable group of normal infants. As a result, the data generated from these studies cannot give a complete picture of the factors contributing to neonatal encephalopathy.

To address these issues, investigators designed a case–control study of all term infants (≥37 weeks or birth weight ≥2,500 g if gestational age was unknown) born in Perth, Western Australia (from June, 1993, through September, 1995), in whom moderate or severe neonatal encephalopathy was diagnosed in the first week of life (23, 24). The study broadly defined neonatal encephalopathy based only on features of abnormal consciousness, tone and reflexes, feeding, respiration, or seizures and did not assume

an intrapartum etiology. A sample of controls was randomly selected from term infants without neonatal encephalopathy in the same study population. Preconceptional, antepartum, intrapartum, newborn, and neonatal variables were all obtained by retrospective review and abstraction of the mothers' and infants' medical records.

A multivariate analysis of 164 cases and 400 controls evaluated the role of preconceptional, antepartum, and intrapartum factors in neonatal encephalopathy (23, 24). The strongest antepartum risk factor for neonatal encephalopathy was fetal growth restriction. There are, however, many different causes of fetal growth restriction, and each may differ in its capacity to cause or predispose a fetus to neonatal encephalopathy. The risk for neonatal encephalopathy also increased with each advancing week of gestation after 39 weeks. Several sociodemographic characteristics were significant risk factors for neonatal encephalopathy (Table 1–1). Significant associations between neonatal encephalopathy and maternal seizures, maternal thyroid disease,

Table 1–1. Preconception Sociodemographic and Maternal Medical Conditions as Statistically Significant Risk Factors for Newborn Encephalopathy

Risk Factor	Reference Group	Unadjusted Risk	Adjusted Odds Ratio (95% confidence interval)
Maternal age (y)	<20	1	1
	20–24	2.37	4.21 (1.10–17.50)
	25–29	1.85	5.91 (1.42–24.54)
	30–34	1.31	6.71 (1.53–29.44)
	>35	1.46	6.01 (1.28–28.15)
Maternal employment	Professional	1	1
	Unskilled manual	2.35	3.84 (1.43–10.28)
	Housewife	3.57	2.48 (1.14–5.39)
	Unemployed	4.47	3.60 (1.10–11.80)
Health insurance	Private	1	1
	Public	2.2	3.46 (1.25–9.59)
Family history of seizures	No	1	—
	Yes	3.10	2.55 (1.31–4.94)
Family history of neurologic disorder	No	1	1
	Yes	2.6	2.73 (1.16–6.41)
Infertility treatment	No	1	1
	Yes	2.23	4.43 (1.12–17.60)

Adapted from Badawi N, Kurinczuk JJ, Keogh JM, Alessandri LM, O'Sullivan F, Burton PR, et al. Antepartum risk factors for newborn encephalopathy: the Western Australian case-control study. BMJ 1998;317:1549–53.

bleeding in pregnancy, an excess of congenital anomalies, and markers of prenatal and perinatal infection were associated with cerebral palsy, supporting the idea of multiple causal pathways leading to neonatal encephalopathy and cerebral palsy (23) (Table 1–2). Of greatest significance, however, was that 70% of cases of neonatal encephalopathy were likely the result of events arising before the onset of labor. Infants with neonatal encephalopathy experienced a more adverse antepartum course than controls, and intrapartum hypoxia was rarely the sole cause of neonatal encephalopathy.

An estimate of the maximal possible contribution of intrapartum hypoxia to neonatal encephalopathy was made using the following criteria (nonspecific with high false-positive pre-dictive values) to indicate intrapartum hypoxia: an abnormal intrapartum cardiotocograph or abnormal fetal heart rate on auscultation or fresh meconium in labor plus both a 1-minute Apgar score less than 3 and a 5-minute Apgar score less than 7. Nineteen percent of case infants (n = 31/164) and 0.5% of controls (n = 2/400) met these criteria. An additional 10% (16 case infants) did not meet these criteria (or the Apgar score was not recorded) but had significant intrapartum events that may have been associated with hypoxia (eg, breech presentation, stuck head), providing a total of 47 case infants (29% of all cases) with any possible evidence of intrapartum hypoxia (24) (Table 1–3). Even using such inexact markers for intrapartum fetal hypoxia, the following notable conclusions were

Table 1–2. Antepartum/Prenatal Maternal Medical and Obstetric and Fetal Characteristics That Are Statistically Significant Risk Factors for Newborn Encephalopathy

Risk Factor	Reference Group	Unadjusted Risk	Adjusted Odds Ratio (95% confidence interval)*
Maternal thyroid disease	No	1	1
	Yes	5.9	9.7 (1.97–47.91)
Preeclampsia	No	1	1
	Severe	3.93	6.30 (2.25–17.62)
Bleeding (moderate or severe)	No	1	1
	Yes	2.32	3.57 (1.30–9.85)
Viral illness	No	1	1
	Yes	2.10	2.97 (1.52–5.80)
Gestational age (wk)	39	1	1
	37	1.44	2.35 (1.11–4.97)
	38	1.10*	1.18 (0.90–1.56)
	40	0.57	1.41 (1.17–1.70)
	41	1.77	3.34 (2.09–5.35)
	42	3.97	13.2 (5.03–34.83)
Centile birth weight	>90th	1	1
	3rd–9th	1.63	4.37 (1.43–13.38)
	<3rd	13.2	38.23 (9.44–154.79)
Abnormal appearance of placenta	Normal	1	1
	Abnormal	3.21	2.07 (1.15–3.73)
Late/no prenatal care	No	1	1
	Yes	15.14*	5.45 (0.47–62.98)

*Not significant increased risk at $P <0.05$

Adapted from Badawi N, Kurinczuk JJ, Keogh JM, Alessandri LM, O'Sullivan F, Burton PR, et al. Antepartum risk factors for newborn encephalopathy: the Western Australian case-control study. BMJ 1998;317:1549–53.

reached regarding all 164 cases of neonatal encephalopathy:

- 69% (113) had only antepartum risk factors

- 25% (40) had both antepartum risk factors and evidence for intrapartum hypoxia

- 4% (7) had evidence of intrapartum hypoxia in the absence of preconceptional or antepartum factors that might also have contributed to neonatal encephalopathy

- 2% (4) had no recognized risk factors for neonatal encephalopathy

The antepartum and intrapartum factors associated with neonatal encephalopathy may act independently of each other, or the antepartum factors may initiate a sequence of events followed by specific intrapartum responses. Alternatively, the imprecise and indirect markers for intrapartum hypoxia currently available may in many cases be the first clinical manifestations of a preexisting injury that has already caused an encephalopathy. To elucidate these different causal pathways it is important that a reliable and readily available assessment of fetal status be possible and that more specific markers of the intrapartum insult be developed (24, 32). It can be said with certainty, however, that the pathway from an intrapartum hypoxic–ischemic injury to subsequent cerebral palsy must progress through neonatal encephalopathy.

Long-Term Neurologic Outcome

Two questions frame the discussion: What proportion of children who have neonatal encephalopathy develop long-term neurologic problems, and, conversely, what proportion of children with long-term neurologic problems had evidence of encephalopathy as neonates?

Most infants with mild to moderate neonatal encephalopathy develop normally (2–4, 33, 34); those with severe neonatal encephalopathy are more likely to sustain long-term neurologic morbidity (2–5, 33–38). The prospectively designed National Collaborative Perinatal Project study monitored approximately 49,000 children from birth to age 7 years. In those infants with an Apgar score of 3 or less at 20 minutes, only 31% survived until age 7 years. However, in those children who had Apgar scores of 0–3 at 20 minutes or more of life and survived, 80% were free of major handicap at early school age (14). Moreover, in children with a 5-minute Apgar score of 3 or less, less than 10% died or developed cerebral palsy or mental retardation (14,

Table 1–3. Intrapartum Conditions as Statistically Significant Risk Factors for Newborn Encephalopathy

Risk Factors	Comparison Group	Unadjusted Odds Risk	Adjusted Odds Ratio (95% confidence interval)
Occipitoposterior position	No	1	1
	Yes	2.97	4.29 (1.74–10.54)
Maternal pyrexia	No	1	1
	Yes	5.34	3.82 (1.44–10.12)
Acute intrapartum event	No	1	1
	Yes	6.80	4.44 (1.30–15.22)
Mode of delivery	Spontaneous	1	1
	Instrumental, vaginal	2.23	2.34 (1.16–4.70)
	Emergency cesarean	2.94	2.17 (1.01–4.64)
	Elective cesarean	0.23	0.17 (0.05–0.56)
General anesthesia	No	1	1
	Yes	4.40*	3.08 (1.16–8.17)

*Not significant increased risk at $P < 0.05$

Adapted from Badawi N, Kurinczuk JJ, Keogh JM, Alessandri LM, O'Sullivan F, Burton PR, et al. Intrapartum risk factors for newborn encephalopathy: the Western Australian case-control study. BMJ 1998;317:1554–8.

39). A review concluded most infants thought to have birth asphyxia did not develop motor or cognitive disabilities unless the asphyxial event was severe and prolonged (39). In the latter instance, infants displayed abnormal neurologic signs as neonates, and the resulting handicaps were generally severe and multiple. In a subsequent reanalysis of the National Collaborative Perinatal Project data, 70% of term or near-term infants either died or developed cerebral palsy if they had a low 5-minute Apgar score, adverse neonatal signs, and seizures (40).

More recently, similar findings (poor neonatal neurologic signs with markers of fetal compromise [eg, abnormal acid–base status at birth]) have been reported in infants with long-term neurologic dysfunction (41). In the same study population, impaired survivors of HIE had a range of developmental handicaps, including severe motor dysfunction, visual impairment, profound developmental delay, and epilepsy (27).

The full range of impairment following an unbiased assessment of neonatal encephalopathy and its subset HIE has not been well-established in a recent and large population-based study. Long-term follow-up studies of children enrolled in large, population-based studies, such as the type of studies described by Badawi et al (22), are needed.

Even though the relative risk for cerebral palsy, and especially spastic quadriplegia, associated with a low 5-minute Apgar score, adverse neonatal signs, and seizures is typically high and statistically significant (ie, infants with these indicators were many times more likely to develop cerebral palsy than were infants without these indicators) (19, 26, 42–44), the proportion of children with cerebral palsy who actually had these indicators is small, that is, less than 10% (26, 27). Analysis of the National Collaborative Perinatal Project data attributed 9% of the cases of cerebral palsy to possible birth asphyxia (45). The calculated fraction of spastic cerebral palsy attributable to birth asphyxia or potential asphyxial events, according to two large population-based studies, was 6–17% for infants of normal birth weight (>2,500 g) (26, 42). In chil-

dren with spastic quadriplegic cerebral palsy, potential asphyxiating events appear to attribute a larger proportion of cases, ranging from 14% (43) to 43% of patients (26). In subsequent studies, it was noted that a certain proportion of the children with spastic cerebral palsy had other risk factors, most often infection or coagulation disorders, that may have contributed to their unfavorable outcome (46, 47).

It is important to understand the concept of attributable fraction in the context of perinatal asphyxia and newborn encephalopathy with long-term neurologic dysfunction. The attributable (or etiologic) fraction represents the proportion of cases in a target population that are attributable to a specific exposure (eg, intrapartum events); it also represents how much of the burden of a specific disease in a population could be eliminated if certain causal factors were eliminated from the group under study (assuming distributions of other risk factors in the population remain unchanged). Attributable fraction is a composite value, based on both the prevalence and relative risk associated with a specific risk factor (48). Because it is a composite value, a risk factor that has a large relative risk for disease but is of low prevalence in the population, it will have a low attributable fraction (49). This is the case when the markers typically used for perinatal asphyxia and cerebral palsy are examined.

Conclusions

- Perinatal asphyxial events clearly can cause newborn neurologic damage and cerebral palsy. The difficulty lies in identifying this causal factor reliably, accurately, and independent of other causal factors.

- The factors used to define perinatal asphyxia are not specific to the disease process leading to neurologic damage. Using a nonspecific marker for perinatal asphyxia falsely identifies a large number of individuals as being exposed to perinatal asphyxia. In turn, the estimates of risk for neurologic damage from perinatal asphyxia identified by such nonspecific markers may include components of risk from other causes also identified by the same marker. Thus, it is not realistic to think that by removing exposure to the nonspecific marker, the risk for disease will necessarily change.

- Neonatal encephalopathy and cerebral palsy rarely are caused by perinatal asphyxia. More often, perinatal asphyxia may be a step in a sequence of events in perhaps more than one causal pathway leading to neonatal encephalopathy and cerebral palsy.

Relationship of Intrapartum Hypoxia and Cerebral Palsy

Cerebral palsy is defined as a chronic neuromuscular disability characterized by abnormal control of movement or posture appearing early in life and not the result of recognized progressive disease (14). The causes of cerebral palsy include developmental malformations, metabolic defects, autoimmune and coagulation disorders, infections, and hypoxia in the fetus and newborn (26, 45, 50).

Neonatal Encephalopathy and Intrapartum Asphyxia

Circulatory Responses

The important circulatory manifestations of asphyxia have been well categorized in experimental studies. These include: 1) a redistribution of cardiac output to preserve blood flow to the more vital organs (ie, brain, myocardium, and adrenal gland) at the expense of flow to less vital organs (ie, parathyroid gland, lung, liver, kidney, intestine, bone marrow, and muscle); 2) loss of cerebral vascular autoregulation resulting in a pressure passive circulation; and 3) eventual diminution in cardiac output with resultant hypotension and ultimately a decrease in cerebral blood flow (51–54). With initial arterial hypoxemia, fetal cerebral vascular resistance can decrease by at least 50% to maintain cerebral blood flow with a minimal decrease in oxygen delivery in an experimental model (55, 56).

Critical to this state is a normal or elevated mean arterial blood pressure. However, with persistent hypoxemia and eventual hypotension, cerebral vascular resistance cannot decrease further, resulting in a marked reduction in cerebral blood flow. The critical ischemic threshold for neuronal necrosis in the developing brain remains unclear. In adults, cerebral blood flow thresholds, below which functional disturbances (electroencephalographic slowing) occur, have been identified. If cerebral blood flow reaches an even lower threshold, ion pump failure occurs (57–59). However, cerebral blood flow values in both preterm and term infants below those that are associated with ion pump failure in adults are associated with subsequent normal neurologic development (60).

Noncirculatory Factors Contributing to Neuronal Preservation

In addition to the circulatory responses described previously, other factors considered potentially important in preserving neuronal integrity during asphyxia include biologic alterations that accompany maturation. Examples include a slower depletion of high-energy compounds during hypoxia–ischemia in the fetus as compared with the term infant or adult (61, 62); the use of alternate energy substrate, the neonatal brain having the capacity to use lactate and ketone bodies for energy production (63, 64); the relative resistance of the fetal and neonatal myocardium to hypoxia–ischemia (65, 66); and the potential protective role of fetal hemoglobin (67, 68).

As a consequence of the previous and other unknown factors, even when asphyxia is prolonged or severe, most newborn infants recover with minimal or no neurologic sequelae. Moreover, some or all of these factors may modulate the neurologic outcome of infants at increased risk for injury (eg, the growth-restricted fetus).

Neuropathology

The neuropathology of intrapartum hypoxic–ischemic cerebral injury may be considered in the context of five basic anatomic subtypes: 1) parasagittal, 2) basal ganglia, 3) periventricular white matter, 4) focal/multifocal, and 5) selective neuronal necrosis. These lesions may overlap; however, the nature of the insult (acute versus intermittent ischemia), the vascular development, and maturation of the brain usually result in a dominant lesion (69). Ischemic necrosis occurs most frequently within border zones between the end branches of the major cerebral blood vessels. These areas are extremely vulnerable to critical decreases in cerebral blood flow. Parasagittal injury is the principal lesion found in fetuses older than 34 weeks of gestation and manifests as spastic quadriplegia. Injury to the basal ganglia follows acute, near-total intrauterine asphyxia and usually involves the thalamus, caudate nucleus, globus palidus, and putamen. Injury to these structures usually is associated with other neuropathologic subtypes (70, 71). Periventricular white matter injury is the principal lesion found in the preterm infant, with the classic manifestation being spastic diplegia (72). Spastic quadriplegia, with accompanying visual and cognitive deficits or defects, may be seen with more severe hypoxic–ischemic injuries.

Focal/multifocal necrosis is characterized by injury to all cellular elements by infarction within a vascular distribution (73). The neurologic manifestations reflect the location and distribution of the lesion. Selective neuronal necrosis is the most common variety of injury observed in HIE (74) and invariably coexists with one or more of those mentioned previously. The intrinsic vulnerability of specific cell types and systems in the developing brain may be the most important factor in determining the final pattern of damage and functional disability. Excitotoxicity caused by overstimulation of excitatory, mainly glutamate, neurotransmitter receptors plays a critical role in these processes (75, 76).

References

1. Fenichel GM. Hypoxic-ischemic encephalopathy in the newborn. Arch Neurol 1983;40:261–6. (Level III)

2. Finer NN, Robertson CM, Richards RT, Pinnell LE, Peters KL. Hypoxic-ischemic encephalopathy in term neonates: perinatal factors and outcome. J Pediatr 1981;98:112–7. (Level II-3)

3. Levene ML, Kornberg J, Williams TH. The incidence and severity of post-asphyxial encephalopathy in full-term infants. Early Hum Dev 1985;11:21–6. (Level III)

4. Low JA, Galbraith RS, Muir DW, Killen HL, Pater EA, Karchmar EJ. The relationship between perinatal hypoxia and newborn encephalopathy. Am J Obstet Gynecol 1985;152:256–60. (Level II-2)

5. Sarnat HB, Sarnat MS. Neonatal encephalopathy following fetal distress. A clinical and electroencephalographic study. Arch Neurol 1976;33:696–705. (Level III)

6. Carter BS, Haverkamp AD, Merenstein GB. The definition of acute perinatal asphyxia. Clin Perinatol 1993;20:287–304. (Level III)

7. Edwards AD, Mehmet H. Apoptosis in perinatal hypoxic-ischemic cerebral damage. Neuropathol Appl Neurobiol 1996;22:494–8. (Level III)

8. Patel J, Edwards AD. Prediction of outcome after perinatal asphyxia. Curr Opin Pediatr 1997;9:128–32. (Level III)

9. Williams CE, Mallard C, Tan W, Gluckman PD. Pathophysiology of perinatal asphyxia. Clin Perinatol 1993;20:305–25. (Level III)

10. Blair E. A research definition for 'birth asphyxia'? Dev Med Child Neurol 1993;35:449–52. (Level III)

11. Goldaber KG, Gilstrap LC 3rd, Leveno KJ, Dax JS, McIntire DD. Pathologic fetal acidemia. Obstet Gynecol 1991;78:1103–7. (Level II-3)

12. Goodwin TM, Belai I, Hernandez P, Durand M, Paul RH. Asphyxial complications in the term newborn with severe umbilical acidemia. Am J Obstet Gynecol 1992;167:1506–12. (Level II-3)

13. Winkler CL, Hauth JC, Tucker JM, Owen J, Bromfield CG. Neonatal complications at term as related to the degree of umbilical artery acidemia. Am J Obstet Gynecol 1991;164:637–41. (Level II-2)

14. Nelson KB, Ellenberg JH. Apgar score as predictors of chronic neurologic disability. Pediatrics 1981;68:36–44. (Level II-2)

15. Ruth VJ, Raivio KO. Perinatal brain damage: predictive value of metabolic acidosis and the Apgar score. BMJ 1988;297:24–7. (Level II-3)

16. Grant A, O'Brien N, Joy MT, Hennessy E, MacDonald D. Cerebral palsy among children born during the Dublin randomised trial of intrapartum monitoring. Lancet 1989;2:1233–6. (Level I)

17. Lumley J. Does continuous intrapartum fetal monitoring predict long-term neurological disorders? Paediatr Perinat Epidemiol 1988;2:299–307. (Level III)

18. Nelson KB, Ellenberg JH. Obstetric complications as risk factors for cerebral palsy or seizure disorders. JAMA 1984;251:1843–8. (Level II-2)

19. Nelson KB, Ellenberg JH. Antecedents of cerebral palsy. I Univariate analysis of risks. Am J Dis Child 1985;139:1031–8. (Level II-2)

20. Nelson KB. Relationship of intrapartum and delivery room events to long-term neurologic outcome. Clin Perinatol 1989;16:995–1007. (Level II-2)

21. Nelson KB, Leviton A. How much of neonatal encephalopathy is due to birth asphyxia? Am J Dis Child 1991;145:1325–31. (Level III)

22. Badawi N, Kurinczuk JJ, Hall D, Field D, Pemberton PJ, Stanley FJ. Newborn encephalopathy in term infants: three approaches to population-based investigation. Semin Neonatol 1997;2:181–8. (Level III)

23. Badawi N, Kurinczuk JJ, Keogh JM, Alessandri LM, O'Sullivan F, Burton PR, et al. Antepartum risk factors for newborn encephalopathy: the Western Australian case-control study. BMJ 1998;317:1549–53. (Level II-2)

24. Badawi N, Kurinczuk JJ, Keogh JM, Alessandri LM, O'Sullivan F, Burton PR, et al. Intrapartum risk factors for newborn encephalopathy: the Western Australian case-control study. BMJ 1998;317:1554–8. (Level II-2)

25. Badawi N, Watson L, Petterson B, Blair E, Slee J, Haan E, et al. What constitutes cerebral palsy? Dev Med Child Neurol 1998;40:520–7. (Level III)

26. Nelson KB, Grether JK. Potentially asphyxiating conditions and spastic cerebral palsy in infants of normal birth weight. Am J Obstet Gynecol 1998;179:507–13. (Level II-2)

27. Yudkin PL, Johnson A, Clover LM, Murphy KW. Assessing the contribution of birth asphyxia to cerebral palsy in term singletons. Paediatr Perinat Epidemiol 1995;9:156–70. (Level II-3)

28. Ergander U, Eriksson M, Zetterstrom R. Severe neonatal asphyxia. Incidence and prediction of outcome in the Stockholm area. Acta Paediatr Scand 1983;72:321–5. (Level III)

29. Thornberg E, Thiringer K, Odeback A, Milsom I. Birth asphyxia: incidence, clinical course and outcome in a Swedish population. Acta Paediatr 1995;84:927–32. (Level II-2)

30. Hull J, Dodd KL. Falling incidence of hypoxic-ischemic encephalopathy in term infants. Br J Obstet Gynaecol 1992;99:386–91. (Level II-3)

31. Nelson KB, Ellenberg JH. The asymptomatic newborn and risk of cerebral palsy. Am J Dis Child 1987;141:1333–5. (Level II-2)

32. Adamson SJ, Alessandri LM, Badawi N, Burton PR, Pemberton PJ, Stanley F. Predictors of neonatal encephalopathy in full-term infants. BMJ 1995;311:598–602. (Level II-2)

33. Robertson C, Finer N. Term infants with hypoxic-ischemic encephalopathy: outcome at 3.5 years. Dev Med Child Neurol 1985;27:473–84. (Level II-3)

34. Robertson CM, Finer NN, Grace MG. School performance of survivors of neonatal encephalopathy associated with birth asphyxia at term. J Pediatr 1989;114:753–60. (Level II-2)

35. Ekert P, Perlman M, Steinlin M, Hao Y. Predicting the outcome of postasphyxial hypoxic-ischemic enceph-alopathy within 4 hours of birth. J Pediatr 1997;131:613–7. (Level II-2)

36. Scott H. Outcome of very severe birth asphyxia. Arch Dis Child 1976;51:712–6. (Level III)

37. Selton D, Andre M. Prognosis of hypoxic-ischaemic encephalopathy in full-term newborns—value of neonatal electroencephalography. Neuropediatrics 1997;28:276–80. (Level II-3)

38. Thomson AJ, Searle M, Russell G. Quality of survival after severe birth asphyxia. Arch Dis Chil 1977;52:620–6. (Level II-2)

39. Paneth N, Stark RI. Cerebral palsy and mental retardation in relation to indicators of perinatal asphyxia. An epidemiologic overview. Am J Obstet Gynecol 1983;147:960–6. (Level III)

40. Ellenberg JH, Nelson KB. Cluster of perinatal events identifying infants at high risk for death or disability. J Pediatr 1988;113:546–52. (Level II-2)

41. Yudkin PL, Johnson A, Clover LM, Murphy KW. Clustering of perinatal markers of birth asphyxia and outcome at age five years. Br J Obstet Gynaecol 1994;101:774–81. (Level II-2)

42. Blair E, Stanley FJ. Intrapartum asphyxia: a rare cause of cerebral palsy. J Pediatr 1988;112:515–9. (Level II-2)

43. Naeye RL, Peters EC, Bartholomew M, Landis JR. Origins of cerebral palsy. Am J Dis Child 1989;143:1154–61. (Level II-2)

44. Torfs CP, van den Berg BJ, Oechsli FW, Cummins S. Prenatal and perinatal factors in the etiology of cerebral palsy. J Pediatr 1990;116:615–9. (Level II-2)

45. Nelson KB, Ellenberg JH. Antecedents of cerebral palsy. Multivariate analysis of risk. N Engl J Med 1986;315:81–6. (Level II-2)

46. Nelson KB, Dambrosia JM, Grether JK, Phillips TM. Neonatal cytokines and coagulation factors in children with cerebral palsy. Ann Neurol 1998;44:665–75. (Level II-2)

47. Nelson KB, Grether JK. Selection of neonates for neuroprotective therapies: one set of criteria applied to a population. Arch Pediatr Adolesc Med 1999;153:393–8. (Level II-2)

48. Rockhill B, Newman B, Weinberg C. Use and misuse of population attributable fractions. Am J Public Health 1998:88:15–9. (Level III)

49. Northridge ME. Public health methods—attributable risk as a link between causality and public health action. Am J Public Health 1995;85:1202–4. (Level III)

50. Grether JK, Nelson KB. Maternal infection and cerebral palsy in infants of normal birth weight. JAMA 1997;278:207–11. (Level II-2)

51. Behrman RE, Lees MH, Petersen EN, De Lannoy CW, Seeds AE. Distribution of the circulation in the normal and asphyxiated fetal primate. Am J Obstet Gynecol 1970;108:956–69. (Animal study)

52. Cohn HE, Sacks EJ, Heymann MA, Rudolf AM. Cardiovascular responses to hypoxemia and acidemia in fetal lambs. Am J Obstet Gynecol 1974;120: 817–24. (Animal study)

53. Peeters LL, Sheldon RE, Jones MD Jr, Makowsk EL, Meschia G. Blood flow to fetal organs as a function of arterial oxygen content. Am J Obstet Gynecol 1979;135:637–46. (Animal study)

54. Sheldon RE, Peeters LL, Jones MD Jr, Makowski EL, Meschia G. Redistribution of cardiac output and oxygen delivery in the hypoxemic fetal lamb. Am J Obstet Gynecol 1979;135:1071–8. (Animal study)

55. Ashwal S, Dale PS, Long LD. Regional cerebral blood flow: studies in the fetal lamb during hypoxia, hypercapnia, acidosis, and hypotension. Pediatr Res 1984; 18:1309–16. (Animal study)

56. Koehler RC, Jones MD Jr, Traystman RJ. Cerebral circulatory response to carbon monoxide and hypoxic hypoxia in the lamb. Am J Physiol 1982;243: H27–H32. (Animal study)

57. Astrup J, Symon L, Branston NM, Lassen NA. Cortical evoked potential and extracellular K+ and H+ at critical levels of brain ischemia. Stroke 1977;8:51–7. (Animal study)

58. Heiss WD, Rosner G. Functional recovery of cortical neurons as related to the degree and duration of ischemia. Ann Neurol 1983;14:294–301. (Animal study)

59. Powers WJ, Grubb RL Jr, Darriet D, Raichle ME. Cerebral blood flow and cerebral metabolic rates of oxygen requirements for cerebral function and viability in humans. J Cereb Blood Flow Metab 1985; 5:600–8. (Level II-2)

60. Altman DI, Powers WJ, Perlman JM, Herscoviteh P, Volpe SL, Volpe JJ. Cerebral blood flow requirement for brain viability in newborn infants is lower than in adults. Ann Neurol 1988;24:218–26. (Level III)

61. Duffy TE, Kohle SJ, Vannucci RC. Carbohydrate and energy metabolism in perinatal rat brain: relation to survival in anoxia. J Neurochem 1975;24:271–6. (Animal study)

62. Holowach-Thurston J, McDougal DB Jr. Effects of ischemia on metabolism of the brain of the newborn mouse. Am J Physiol 1964;216:348–52b. (Animal study)

63. Cremer JE. Substrate utilization and brain development. J Cereb Blood Flow Metab 1982;2:394–407. (Level III)

64. Yager JY, Heitjan DF, Towfighi J, Vannuci RC. Effect of insulin-induced and fasting hypoglycemia on perinatal hypoxic-ischemic brain damage. Pediatr Res 1992;31:138–42. (Animal study)

65. Dawes GS, Mott JC, Shelley HJ. The importance of cardiac glycogen for the maintenance of life in foetal lambs and newborn animals during anoxia. J Physiol 1959;146:516–38. (Animal study)

66. Wells RJ, Friedman WF, Sobel BE. Increased oxidative metabolism in the fetal and newborn lamb heart. Am J Physiol 1972;222:1488–93. (Animal study)

67. Ramaekers VT, Daniels H, Casaer P. Brain oxygen transport related to levels of fetal haemoglobin in stable preterm infants. J Dev Physiol 1992;17:209–13. (Level II-3)

68. Wimberly PD. A review of oxygen delivery in the neonate? J Clin Lab Invest 1982;160(supple):114–8. (Level III)

69. Volpe JJ. Neurology of the newborn. 4th ed. Philadelphia (PA): WB Saunders; 2001. (Level III)

70. Myers RE. Four patterns of perinatal brain damage and their conditions of occurrence in primates. Adv Neurol 1975;10:223–34. (Animal study)

71. Pasternak JF, Garey MT. The syndrome of acute near-total intrauterine asphyxia in the term infant. Pediatr Neurol 1998;18:391–8. (Level III)

72. Chen CH, Shen WC, Wang TM, Chi CS. Cerebral magnetic resonance imaging of preterm infants after corrected age of one year. Zhonghua Min Guo Xiao Er Ke Yi Xue Hui Za Zhi 1995;36:261–5. (Level III)

73. Perlman JM, Rollins NK, Evans D. Neonatal stroke: clinical characteristics and cerebral blood flow velocity measurements. Pediatr Neurol 1994;11:281–4. (Level III)

74. Scott RJ, Hegyi L. Cell death in perinatal hypoxic-ischaemic brain injury. Neuropathol Appl Neurobiol 1997;23:307–14. (Level II-2)

75. Johnston MV, Trescher WH, Ishida A, Nakajima W. Neurobiology of hypoxic-ischemic injury in the developing brain. Pediatr Res 2001;49:735–41. (Level III)

76. McDonald JW, Johnston MV. Physiological and pathophysiological roles of excitatory amino acids during central nervous system development. Brain Res Rev 1990;15:41–70. (Animal study)

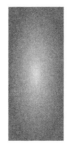

CHAPTER 2

MATERNAL CONDITIONS

Third-Trimester Maternal Bleeding as a Risk Factor

Maternal shock from hemorrhage caused by placenta previa or abruption can result in impaired oxygen delivery to the fetus. Despite this, third-trimester bleeding is rarely associated with neonatal hypoxic–ischemic encephalopathy (HIE). A significant association has been reported between neuronal necrosis, white-matter gliosis or necrosis, and pathologically diagnosed placental abruption (1). Early research demonstrated an association between maternal bleeding in pregnancy and cerebral palsy, but most of those studies were flawed by their failure to consider confounding variables such as the effect of low birth weight. Review of the studies that have controlled for fetal growth restriction suggests an association, if present, is not very strong and is limited to term pregnancies.

The literature is considered inconsistent with respect to findings on the relationship between third-trimester bleeding and neonatal encephalopathy. In a case–control study among Western Australian women and their term infants (89 cases, 89 matched controls), vaginal bleeding was associated with neonatal encephalopathy (odds ratio [OR], 5; 95% confidence interval [CI], 1.5–17.3) (2). However, this study did not control for underlying maternal or pregnancy-related conditions that may have contributed to the bleeding. In another case–control study (164 cases, 412 randomly selected controls) conducted by the same group, a significant association between moderate-to-severe antepartum vaginal bleeding and newborn encephalopathy was noted (OR, 3.57; 95% CI, 1.30–9.85) (3). This association was independent of maternal hypertension or fever. In a prospective U.S. study that followed a cohort of 42,704 mothers who gave birth to infants weighing more than 2,500 g, placenta previa and placental abruption were evaluated as distinct factors (4). Placenta previa was determined to be a risk factor for cerebral palsy for infants weighing more than 2,500 g (OR, 6; 95% CI, 1.9–18.8). Although placental abruption carried an increased risk for fetal death in the first year of life, the risk of cerebral palsy in the survivors was not elevated. This study did not control for maternal or pregnancy factors that may have contributed to placenta previa or abruption. A case–control study of 46 infants, weighing more than 2,500 g, with unexplained spastic cerebral palsy and 378 randomly selected controls from the California Birth Defects Monitoring Program demonstrated that neither placental abruption (OR, 4.3; 95% confidence interval, 0.65–39) nor previa (OR, 2.8; 95% CI, 0.52–25) was associated with a significantly increased risk for cerebral palsy (5). A subgroup analysis found placental abruption (OR, 11.0; 95% CI, 1.6–103) and placenta previa (OR, 7.4; 95% CI, 1.3–66) were associated with elevated risks for the cerebral palsy subtype spastic quadriplegia. This study evaluated placenta previa and abruption as univariate risk factors.

The only published paper to evaluate the relationship between third-trimester maternal bleeding and HIE in preterm infants was a Danish case–control study (6). In this study, neither placenta previa (OR, 0.26; 95% CI, 0.1–1.1) nor abruption (OR, 0.97; 95% CI, 0.61–1.55) was a significant predictor of cerebral palsy.

Calculated risks for neonates developing cerebral palsy after delivery from mothers with placenta previa or abruption are problematic and likely represent unstable estimates. Moreover, placental abruption does not necessarily arise de novo but most often in association with underlying disease states such as hypertension, coagulopathy, substance abuse, uterine overdistension, or infection. Intervention during labor cannot reverse these underlying causes of bleeding or other antecedent events that may have caused damage to the fetus.

Conclusions

- Third-trimester placental bleeding is often associated with a chronic and long-standing underlying condition that may have resulted in fetal injury antedating clinical bleeding.

- Third-trimester placental bleeding is rarely associated with neonatal HIE.

Maternal Trauma During Pregnancy

The only published systematic analysis of maternal trauma and cerebral palsy was a population-based study from the Maternal and Child Health Research Database in Western Australia (7). This study examined 286,745 births and 770 cases of cerebral palsy, two of which were associated with mothers who sustained trauma during pregnancy. This study did not find a significant relationship between the two variables (unadjusted

relative risk [RR], 1.4; 95% CI, 0.3–5.8). Maternal trauma as a predecessor of neonatal HIE is extremely rare, and estimates of risk for a neonate developing cerebral palsy after delivery from a mother who sustains trauma would be highly prone to error.

Conclusion

- Maternal trauma as a predecessor of neonatal HIE is extremely rare.

Inflammation, Infection, Coagulation Abnormalities, and Autoimmune Disorders

Inflammatory Mechanisms Linked to Neonatal Encephalopathy and Brain Damage

Epidemiology

Although preterm or low-birth-weight (<2,500 g) infants experience at least eightfold greater risks of cerebral palsy than term newborns (8), children born at or near term continue to represent more than one half of children with cerebral palsy. Infection/inflammation and thrombosis/thrombophilias are increasingly recognized as causes of preterm birth and low birth weight as well as periventricular white-matter damage and subsequent cerebral palsy.

Infections and Other Initiators of Inflammation

Intrauterine exposure to infection is associated with a risk of cerebral palsy in the term and near-term infant (9,10) and is probably the most common antecedent of low Apgar scores and other indicators of neonatal depression (11–14). Evidence linking infection to cerebral palsy is summarized as follows:

- Intrauterine exposure to maternal or placental infection is associated with hypotension, neonatal seizures, need for intubation, meconium aspiration syndrome, multiorgan involvement, chorioamnionitis, amniotic fluid infection, preterm delivery, and a clinical diagnosis of HIE or neonatal encephalopathy (3, 12, 13, 15). Intrauterine infection and inflammation are similarly linked to intraventricular hemorrhage, white-matter damage, periventricular leukomalacia, bronchopulmonary dysplasia, and cerebral palsy in the fetus and newborn (16–18).

- The fetal–neonatal inflammatory response (19) is comparable to the systemic inflammatory response syndrome described in adults and is probably mediated in part by widespread endothelial injury (20).

- It has been hypothesized that intrauterine exposure to infection causes fetal overproduction of cytokines, leading to cellular damage in the fetal brain. One study found increased levels of inflammatory cytokines in the amniotic fluid of infants with white-matter lesions and found that these cytokines were overexpressed in the brains of infants who have periventricular leukomalacia (21).

- Chorioamnionitis in very-low-birth-weight infants is significantly associated with an increase in periventricular leukomalacia ($P = 0.001$) (22). In a recent meta-analysis, clinical chorioamnionitis has a RR of 1.9 (95% CI, 1.4–2.5) for development of cerebral palsy in preterm infants and a RR of 4.7 (95% CI, 1.3–16.2) in term infants (23).

- Children exposed to infection in utero, who also had potentially asphyxiating obstetric complications, were at much higher risk for cerebral palsy than those with only one or no other risk factors (9, 24)

- Available studies of term infants include little information about cerebral palsy risk associated with intrauterine infection before the peripartum period or on the contribution of extrauterine infection.

Several biologic pathways of intrauterine infection and inflammation leading to fetal and perinatal brain damage have been documented by research in the past 20 years. These "pathobiologic pathways" clarify the multiple links between maternal and perinatal inflammation, cerebral palsy, and other closely associated complications (25). To put these pathways in perspective, three newer concepts related to infection/inflammation and perinatal brain damage should be recognized:

1 Inflammatory responses of both the perinate and the mother to ascending or blood-borne intrauterine infections are mediated by each individual's genetically controlled inflammatory process (26).

2. Intrauterine infection may precede pregnancy or be established very early in pregnancy. Endometrial or decidual infection may remain clinically unrecognized and may even persist from one pregnancy to the next (27).

3. The end results of infections and inflammatory processes in the maternal and fetal compartments include not only abscess formation, cellulitis, thrombosis, embolization, ischemia and infarction, but also cell damage from reactive oxygen species and other damaging molecules, altered immune recognition, and apoptosis or programmed cell death. It is likely that noninfectious causes of inflammation, such as immune perturbations or abnormalities between the fetus and mother, can also play determining roles in fetal outcomes. These brain-damaging mechanisms may persist and cause damage after the original harmful processes have been removed or corrected (21, 27).

Preterm and Low-Birth-Weight Births

Infection/inflammation is the most commonly identified cause of preterm birth at the lowest viable gestational ages. Studies document increased fetal cytokines measured by amniocentesis and cordocentesis in association with preterm labor or premature rupture of membranes and positive amniotic fluid cultures (28, 29). In one study, fetal interleukin (IL)-6 levels were elevated in fetuses delivering within 48 hours, while maternal levels were normal (29). Microorganisms enter upper reproductive tract tissues primarily by ascending through the cervix or, less commonly, by way of the maternal blood stream. The most common microorganisms found in intrauterine infection and inflammation are bacterial-vaginosis-associated microbes (including anaerobes, genital mycoplasmas, and *Gardnerella vaginalis*) and endogenous vaginal microflora of varying potential virulence. Treatment of these infections antenatally has not been shown to prevent preterm labor or premature rupture of membranes.

Elevated cytokine concentrations in amniotic fluid (21) and umbilical cord blood (30) are associated with white-matter damage and cerebral palsy. Another study linked increased IL-6 levels at cordocentesis with doubling the risk of newborns developing combined clinical markers of "severe neonatal morbidity" (78% versus 30% (19). This comprehensive multiorgan endpoint was defined as the presence of respiratory distress syndrome, pneumonia, bronchopulmonary dysplasia, suspected or proven neonatal sepsis, intraventricular hemorrhage, periventricular leukomalacia, or necrotizing enterocolitis. Martinez and colleagues described similarly increased risks as well as periventricular leukomalacia in neonates with positive amniotic fluid cultures or increased IL-6 concentrations (31).

Term and Near-Term Births

Research has shown an association between ultrasound findings of periventricular leukomalacia and markers of intrauterine infection, including clinical chorioamnionitis, elevated maternal C-reactive protein (CRP), and recovery of placental microbes (32). A case–control study using blood samples obtained shortly after birth of term or near-term newborns has demonstrated strong associations among cerebral palsy, increased neonatal cytokines, and evidence of neonatal thrombophilia (33, 34). In 31 children with unexplained cerebral palsy born at or near term, there were marked elevations in panels of blood levels of cytokines and chemokines when compared with control children. All affected children had significant colinear increases in proinflammatory cytokines (eg, IL-1, tumor necrosis factor-a) over those found in healthy babies. Proinflammatory cytokines were higher in children of mothers with clinically recognized perinatal infection, children with spastic diplegia,

and children with 5-minute Apgar scores below 6 (34). Increased levels of IL-9 or IL-11 distinguished children with cerebral palsy from control children in this series. In this population-based study there also appeared to be a strong relationship between proinflammatory cytokine activation and thrombophilia, including genetically mediated conditions. Although each child with otherwise unexplained cerebral palsy demonstrated cytokine increases, 65% (20 of 31) demonstrated evidence of one or more perinatal thrombophilias. This suggests thrombophilia is associated with inflammatory activation in many children who will manifest cerebral palsy. Conversely, evidence of inflammation also is common in the presence of thrombophilia.

Conclusions

- Clinical and subclinical reproductive tract infection is a cause of reproductive loss and preterm birth, especially at the earliest viable gestational ages.

- The presence of intrauterine infection and inflammatory cytokines are associated with the increased risk for the development of cerebral palsy in both preterm and term infants.

Infection/Inflammation-Linked Complications of Pregnancy and Cerebral Palsy

Some studies (4, 35), but not all (36, 37), show a connection between premature or prolonged preterm rupture of membranes and cerebral palsy. A study of premature preterm rupture of membranes at or before 33 weeks of gestation noted an increased risk of cerebral palsy (adjusted OR, 4.3; 95% CI, 1.6–11.8) (38). These findings were consistent with those in a similar low-birth-weight (<1,500 g) population (39).

Chorioamnionitis: Clinical and Histologic

Associations among histologic and clinical chorioamnionitis and white-matter lesions, echolucency, and periventricular leukomalacia appear complex and not completely understood. This is possibly because of differences in populations studied, study size, or in how studies were conducted (25, 40, 41). An association between chorioamnionitis and periventricular leukomalacia also has been noted in mothers with findings suggestive of bacterial vaginosis (40).

Multiple studies using univariate analyses show increased risks of cerebral palsy in the presence of clinically defined chorioamnionitis in preterm or low-birth-weight (<2,500 g) newborns (4, 35, 36, 42–44).

Bacterial Causes of Cerebral Palsy and Perinatal Encephalopathy

Common aerobic bacterial pathogens can cause invasive disease of each of the fetus's or newborn's organ systems, including the central nervous system. Both single isolate and combined infections can cause lethal intrauterine infection/inflammation and fetal infection. Microorganisms, such as a group B streptococci (45, 46); enteric bacteria, including *Escherichia coli* (especially K-1 serotype), *Klebsiella*, and *Proteus* species; oropharyngeal microbes, including unconjugated *Haemophilus* species and, less commonly group A streptococcus and *Staphylococcus aureus*; as well as less common enteropathogens *Listeria monocytogenes* and certain *Salmonella* species can cause fetal and newborn sepsis, including meningitis, meningoencephalitis, cerebritis, and vasculitis (47). Anaerobes and genital mycoplasmas are commonly isolated in the amniotic fluid from cases of clinical chorioamnionitis but are less commonly isolated from neonatal blood or cerebrospinal fluid cultures than more common aerobic pathogens. One study suggested chorioamnionitis caused by coagulase-negative staphylococci may be an important mediator of cerebral palsy (48).

As in adult sepsis, systemic inflammatory responses occur in fetal and neonatal infections (19). These complex sets of reactions involve a "cascade" of cytokines, chemokines, coagulation factors, kinases, and myriad other cellular responses that are understood to be more important in determining the organism's ultimate survival and possible sequelae than the original microbial infection. Systemic as well as local inflammatory responses can cause direct cell death (necrosis) as well as inducing the process of programmed cell death or apoptosis. Apoptosis as well as alteration of cell antigenicity and host immune responsiveness can foster ongoing brain and other cell damage. Local secondary damage from reactive oxygen species and proteolytic enzymes released during phagocytic killing of microorganisms can perpetuate cell damage after the original infection (49).

Viral and Protozoal Causes of Cerebral Palsy and Encephalopathy

Viral and protozoal infections during pregnancy are well described as less common or geographically limited causes of cerebral palsy and encephalopathy. Congenital nonbacterial infections were considered causative in 6 of 84 cases of cerebral palsy in one large U.S. population-based cohort study (13). The most important nonbacterial vertical infections causing brain damage include infections caused by cytomegalovirus, enteroviruses, human herpes viruses 1 and 2, varicella–zoster virus, and rubella, as well as toxoplasmosis and congenital malaria.

Fetal and Maternal Thrombosis and Coagulopathy

Analyses of placental pathology have suggested a relationship between various thrombotic placental lesions, stillbirth, organ thrombosis, and early neonatal death (50). In another review, fetal placental vessels showed obvious thrombi in 11 of 15 children with well-documented cerebral palsy (51).

Investigators have suggested maternal or fetal coagulopathies or both constitute important causes of lethal or disabling thrombosis and cerebral palsy before birth. They have proposed that identifiable maternal coagulation abnormalities may be transmittable across the placenta or, alternatively, that the fetus can manifest its own coagulation disorders (50).

These findings are supported by a 1994 study of 98 autopsies (1). This study correlated brain and placental pathology. Most brain abnormalities fell into one of three categories, each of which was linked to placental findings: 1) germinal matrix/intraventricular hemorrhage, linked to funisitis; 2) white-matter gliosis/necrosis, linked to placental chronic vascular conditions, umbilical cord problems, old placental infarcts, and meconium exposure; and 3) neuronal necrosis, linked to surface vessel thrombosis and infarction/abruption (1). This investigator concluded that different types of brain injury may occur remote from parturition (1).

In another study, investigators analyzed dried and frozen heel-stick filter paper blood samples obtained from newborns (33). This case–control study compared 53 analytes in blood samples obtained from 31 children with spastic cerebral palsy of unknown cause with those of 65 control children. Another eight had elevated concentrations of the translational product of factor V Leiden mutation. There were elevated concentrations of protein-C antigen in 11 children. Seven children with cerebral palsy had increased concentrations of protein-C antigen. Elevations of the factor V Leiden mutation product and protein-C or protein-S concentrations were not related to clinical indicators of exposure to maternal infection and were not correlated with inflammatory cytokines (34). Twenty of the 31 children with cerebral palsy of unknown origin had one or more abnormalities of coagulation. All of the children with cerebral palsy of unknown origin also demonstrated increased cytokines, which suggests a relationship between inflammatory activation and perinatal coagulopathies. Several children demonstrated multiple coagulation-related abnormalities. Four children (4/31, or 13%) demonstrated antiphospholipid antibody in titers of 1:100 or greater. Smaller numbers of children with cerebral palsy had significantly increased concentrations of antibody to antithrombin III, to a translational product of the factor V Leiden mutation, and to protein C and protein S.

The authors of the study concluded that both intrauterine infection and disorders of coagulation were risk factors for spastic cerebral palsy in children born at or near term (24). They further observed that low Apgar scores, need for resuscitation, and seizures were nonspecific indicators of perinatal or neonatal illness and did not identify clinical or pathophysiologic processes.

Increasing evidence shows that both maternal and fetal thrombophilias may damage the developing embryo and fetus. Maternal antibodies to coagulation factors, phospholipids, and many other potential maternal or fetal antigens are actively and passively transported across the placenta. The presence of maternal antibody to cardiolipin as a risk factor for nonreassuring fetal status or fetal death in mothers with systemic lupus erythematosus is well described (52). Similarly, placental (fetal compartment) correlates of maternal lupus and phospholipid antibody syndrome (thrombosis, infarction) have been characterized (53).

Evidence that a child's genome may directly predispose to thrombotic conditions and cerebral palsy before and after birth has been reported. Investigators have described heterozygosity for factor V Leiden mutation in three children with cerebral palsy (54). One child had extensive placental thrombosis, and all three had evidence of peripartum ischemic or hemorrhagic stroke. Other researchers have demonstrated that fetal carriers of factor V Leiden mutation are prone to death and placental infarction (55). A case analysis of eight children with elevated levels of the translational product of the factor V Leiden mutation and a diagnosis of cerebral palsy revealed the following clinical symptoms in a variety of combinations: low birth weight, fetal distress, respiratory problems, intrauterine growth restriction, neonatal seizures, and a diagnosis of birth asphyxia. Neuroimaging studies, available on four of the children, indicated cerebral infarction or intraventricular hemorrhage or both (56).

Conclusions

- The presence of coagulation disorders in the mother (eg, antithrombin-III deficiency, abnormalities of protein C or protein S, and the factor V Leiden mutation) may be associated with the origin of cerebral palsy in the child.

- Maternal clinical chorioamnionitis, severe histologic chorioamnionitis, and histologic funisitis are associated with cerebral palsy. Mild histologic chorioamnionitis does not appear to be associated with cerebral palsy.

Autoimmune Disorders

Data are scant that relate autoimmune disorders to cerebral palsy. No studies have adequately addressed the association between autoimmune disorders in the mother and cerebral palsy in the child.

Thyroid Disorders (Hypothyroidism) and Cerebral Palsy

Observational studies have shown an association between transient low thyroid hormone and abnormal neurologic development in the preterm infant (57–62). There is considerable evidence that severe thyroid dysfunction in the mother has an adverse effect on fetal neurodevelopment (63, 64). A retrospective cohort study found a significant relationship between maternal thyroid disease of any type and neonatal encephalopathy (62). A follow-up of this study did not allow for a conclusion on cerebral palsy, and it is far less clear whether maternal thyroid disease is related to cerebral palsy.

Conclusions

- Maternal thyroid disease is a risk factor for abnormal neurodevelopment in the neonate.
- Evidence that thyroid disorders are related to cerebral palsy are conflicting and require further investigation.

Epilepsy and Antiepileptic Drugs

Various investigators have suggested a link between epilepsy (ie, seizures) in the mother and an increased risk of cerebral palsy in the offspring, and the presence of mental retardation in the mother may suggest an association with cere-

bral palsy in the newborn (63–65). A univariate analysis of risks for cerebral palsy from the National Collaborative Perinatal Project data identified maternal mental retardation and seizures as risk factors for cerebral palsy in the offspring (63). A multivariate analysis of the same data (64) revealed the same risk factors, but the 95% CIs both crossed one, thus failing to achieve statistical significance. Other investigators demonstrated a family history of seizures or neurologic disorders—defined as any mention of these conditions in up to a second-degree relative of the child—was associated with a 2.5-fold increase in relative risk for neonatal encephalopathy in term infants (3). No determination was made as to the likelihood of cerebral palsy in the affected newborns. There are no data to support that the use of antiepileptic drugs in the mother has any association with the development of cerebral palsy in the offspring.

Conclusion

- The link between maternal epilepsy or mental retardation and cerebral palsy in the offspring may be more of an association than direct causation.

Environmental Factors, Chemicals, Alcohol Use, and Illicit Drug Use

Environmental Factors

Few studies address the association of environmental factors with neurologic development, especially with regard to neonatal encephalopathy and subsequent neurologic dysfunction. However, one of the best-known environmental toxins, methylmercury, has been shown to cause damage to the developing brain. Cerebral atrophy, cerebral palsy, mental retardation, spasticity, seizures, and blindness have all been reported to be associated with exposure to high concentrations of organic mercury during pregnancy (66). However, no increases in teratogenic or adverse pregnancy effects were found in two reports of occupational metallic mercury exposure among dental workers (67, 68).

Lead exposure has been posited as a potential teratogenic agent, and reports have associated lowered IQ and mental retardation with levels of lead in blood (69, 70). However, two large studies found no increase in major congenital anomalies among newborns with elevated levels of lead in cord blood (69, 71). If maternal lead exposure is associated with adverse neurologic development and cerebral palsy, the level and degree of lead exposure resulting in such damage is unknown.

The association of maternal hyperthermia (via hot tubs or saunas, for example) with adverse fetal neurologic development is unclear. However, an association between maternal heat exposure and neural tube defects has been reported (72).

Chemicals

No scientific data support an association of neonatal neurologic maldevelopment or damage from maternal occupational exposure to organic solvents (eg, painters, gas station attendants), general chemicals (eg, hairdressers, dry cleaning workers), or various pesticides (with the exception of methylmercury) (73).

Alcohol and Illicit Drug Exposure

The adverse fetal effects of maternal alcohol exposure are well known. Fetal alcohol syndrome, which includes fetal growth restriction, craniofacial anomalies, and neurologic dysfunction, was first described in 1973 (74). Approximately 4% of offspring of alcoholic mothers have fetal alcohol syndrome (74–76). The effect of sporadic or low levels of alcohol exposure on fetal neurologic development is unclear, and what constitutes a "safe" level of maternal alcohol intake during pregnancy is unknown. However, it seems reasonable to conclude from available evidence that moderate to heavy maternal alcohol use may result in neonatal neurologic dysfunction, behavioral abnormalities, and cognitive dysfunction. Finally, maternal alcoholism is one of the leading preventable causes of fetal neurodevelopmental disorders (77).

The effects of maternal cocaine exposure on fetal neurologic development are less clear than the effects of alcohol to the developing fetus. However, there have been numerous reports of maternal cocaine use and fetal brain damage (78–83). Two reports of maternal cocaine exposure and adverse fetal effects suggest maternal cocaine abuse is associated with a decrease in newborn head circumference (84, 85). The potential effects of other illicit substances such as methamphetamines and marijuana on fetal neurologic development are unknown.

Conclusions

- There are few data regarding the association of environmental factors, newborn encephalopathy, and subsequent neurologic dysfunction.

- Cerebral palsy, cerebral atrophy, and neurologic dysfunction have been associated with maternal exposure to concentrations of organic mercury exposure.

- Moderate to heavy maternal alcohol use may result in neonatal neurologic dysfunction, behavioral abnormalities, and cognitive dysfunction.

- There is no known relationship between alcohol consumption and cerebral palsy.

- Until more data are available regarding the effects of occasional, light alcohol consumption on the developing fetus, pregnant women should avoid alcohol altogether.

- Maternal cocaine use may affect fetal neurologic development.

References

1. Grafe MR. The correlation of prenatal brain damage with placental pathology. J Neuropathol Exp Neurol 1994;53:407–15. (Level III)

2. Adamson SJ, Alessandri LM, Badawi N, Burton PR, Pemberton PJ, Stanley F. Predictors of neonatal encephalopathy in full-term infants. BMJ 1995;311: 598–602. (Level II-2)

3. Badawi N, Kurinczuk JJ, Keogh JM, Alessandri LM, O'Sullivan F, Burton PR, et al. Antepartum risk factors for newborn encephalopathy: the Western Australian case-control study. BMJ 1998;317: 1549–53. (Level II-2)

4. Nelson KB, Ellenberg JH. Obstetric complications as risk factors for cerebral palsy or seizure disorders. JAMA 1984;251:1843–8. (Level II-2)

5. Nelson KB, Grether JK. Potentially asphyxiating conditions and spastic cerebral palsy in infants of normal birth weight. Am J Obstet Gynecol 1998;179: 507–13. (Level II-2)

6. Topp M, Langhoff-Roos J, Uldall P. Preterm birth and cerebral palsy. Predictive value of pregnancy complications, mode of delivery, and Apgar scores. Acta Obstet Gynecol Scand 1997;76:843–8. (Level II-2)

7. Gilles MT, Blair E, Watson L, Badawi N, Alessandri L, Dawes V, et al. Trauma in pregnancy and cerebral palsy: is there a link? Med J Aust 1996;164:500–1. (Level II-2)

8. Topp M, Uldall P, Langhoff-Roos J. Trend in cerebral palsy birth prevalence in eastern Denmark: birth-year period 1979-86. Paediatr Perinat Epidemiol 1997;11: 451–60. (Level II-2)

9. Nelson KB, Willoughby RE. Infection, inflammation and the risk of cerebral palsy. Curr Opin Neurol 2000;13:133–9. (Level III)

10. Eastman NJ, DeLeon M. The etiology of cerebral palsy. Am J Obstet Gynecol 1955;69:950–61. (Level III)

11. Alexander JM, McIntire DM, Leveno KJ. Chorioamnionitis and the prognosis for term infants. Obstet Gynecol 1999;94:274–8. (Level II-2)

12. Badawi N, Kurinczuk JJ, Keogh JM, Alessandri LM, O'Sullivan F, Burton PR, et al. Intrapartum risk factors for newborn encephalopathy: the Western Australian case-control study. BMJ 1998;317: 1554–8. (Level II-2)

13. Grether JK, Nelson KB. Maternal infection and cerebral palsy in infants of normal birth weight. JAMA 1997;278:207–11. (Level II-2)

14. Perlman JM. Maternal fever and neonatal depression: preliminary observations. Clin Pediatr 1999;38: 287–91. (Level II-2)

15. Keogh JM, Badawi N, Kurinczuk JJ, Pemberton PJ, Stanley FJ. Group B streptococcus infection, not birth asphyxia. Aust N Z J Obstet Gynaecol 1999;39: 108–10. (Level III)

16. Vigneswaran R. Infection and preterm birth: evidence of a common causal relationship with bronchopulmonary dysplasia and cerebral palsy. J Paediatr Child Health 2000;36:293–6. (Level III)

17. Watterberg KL, Demers LM, Scott SM, Murphy S. Chrioamnionitis and early lung inflammation in infants in whom bronchopulmonary dysplasia develops. Pediatrics 1996;97:210–5. (Level II-2)

18. Bejar R, Wozniak P, Allard M, Benirschke K, Vaucher Y, Coen R, et al. Antenatal origin of neurologic damage in newborn infants. I. Preterm infants. Am J Obstet Gynecol 1988;159:357–63. (Level II-2)

19. Gomez R, Romero R, Ghezzi F, Yoon BH, Mazor M, Berry SM. The fetal inflammatory response syndrome. Am J Obstet Gynecol 1998;197:194–202. (Level II-2)

20. Garcia-Fernandez N, Montes R, Purroy A, Rocha E. Hemostatic disturbances in patients with systemic inflammatory response syndrome (SIRS) and associated acute renal failure (ARF). Thromb Res 2000; 100:19–25. (Level II-2)

21. Yoon BH, Romero R, Kim CJ, Koo JN, Choe G, Syn HC, et al. High expression of tumor necrosis factor-alpha and interleukin-6 in periventricular leukomalacia. Am J Obstet Gynecol 1997;177:406–11. (Level II-2)

22. Alexander JM, Gilstrap LC, Cox SM, McIntire DM, Leveno KJ. Clinical chorioamnionitis and the prognosis for very low birth weight infants. Obstet Gynecol 1998;91:725–9. (Level II-2)

23. Wu YW, Colford JM Jr. Chorioamnionitis as a risk factor for cerebral palsy. A meta-analysis. JAMA 2000;284:1417–24. (Meta-analysis)

24. Nelson KB, Grether JK. Causes of cerebral palsy. Curr Opin Pediatr 1999;11:487–91. (Level III)

25. Dammann O, Durum SK, Leviton A. Modification of the infection-associated risks of preterm birth and white matter in the preterm newborn by polymorphisms in the tumor necrosis factor–locus? Pathogenesis 1999;1:171–7. (Level III)

26. Eschenbach DA. Amniotic fluid infection and cerebral palsy [editorial]. Focus on the fetus. JAMA 1997; 278:247–8. (Level III)

27. Goldenberg RL, Hauth JC, Andrews WW. Intrauterine infection and preterm delivery. N Engl J Med 2000;342:1500–7. (Level III)

28. Romero R, Brody DT, Oyarzun E, Mazor M, Wu YR, Hobbins JC, et al. Infection and labor. III. Interleukin-1: a signal for the onset of parturition. Am J Obstet Gynecol 1989; 160:1117–23. (Level II-2)

29. Romero R, Gomez R, Ghezzi F, Yoon BH, Mazor M, Edwin SS, et al. A fetal systemic inflammatory response is followed by the spontaneous onset of preterm parturition. Am J Obstet Gynecol 1998;179: 186–93. (Level II-2)

30. Yoon BH, Romero R, Yang SH, Jun JK, Kim IO, Choi JH, et al. Interleukin-6 concentrations in umbilical cord plasma are elevated in neonates with white matter lesions associated with periventricular leukomalacia. Am J Obstet Gynecol 1996;174:1433–40. (Level II-2)

31. Martinez E, Figueroa R, Garry D, Visintainer P, Patel K, Verma U, et al. Elevated amniotic fluid interleukin-6 as a predictor of neonatal periventricular leukomalacia and intraventricular hemorrhage. J Matern Fetal Investig 1998;8:101–7. (Level II-2)

32. Baud O, Emilie D, Pelletier E, Lacaze-Masmonteil T, Zupan V, Fernandez H, et al. Amniotic fluid concentrations of interleukin-1beta, interleukin-6 and

TNF-alpha in chorioamnionitis before 32 weeks of gestation: histological associations and neonatal outcome. Br J Obstet Gynaecol 1999;106:72–7. (Level II-2)

33. Grether JK, Nelson KB, Dambrosia JM, Phillips TM. Interferons and cerebral palsy. J Pediatr 1999;134: 324–32. (Level II-2)

34. Nelson KB, Dambrosia JM, Grether JK, Phillips TM. Neonatal cytokines and coagulation factors in children with cerebral palsy. Ann Neurol 1998;44: 665–75. (Level II-2)

35. Spinillo A, Capuzzo E, Orcesi S, Stronati M, Di Mario M, Fazzi E. Antenatal and delivery risk factors simultaneously associated with neonatal death and cerebral palsy in preterm infants. Early Hum Dev 1997; 48:81–91. (Level II-2)

36. O'Shea TM, Klinepeter KL, Meis PJ, Dillard RG. Intrauterine infection and the risk of cerebral palsy in very low-birthweight infants. Paediatr Perinat Epidemiol 1998;12:72–83. (Level II-2)

37. Kurki T, Hallman M, Zilliacus R, Teramo K, Ylikorkala O. Premature rupture of membranes: effect of penicillin prophylaxis and long-term outcome of the children. Am J Perinatol 1992;9:11–6. (Level II-2)

38. Burguet A, Monnet F, Pauchard JY, Roth P, Fromentin C, Dalphin ML,et al. Some risk factors for cerebral palsy in very premature infants: importance of premature rupture of membranes and monochorionic twin placentation. Biol Neonate 1999;75:177–86. (Level II-2)

39. Dammann O, Leviton A. Infection remote from the brain, neonatal white matter damage, and cerebral palsy in the preterm infant. Semin Pediatr Neurol 1998;5:190–201. (Level III)

40. Spinillo A, Capuzzo E, Stronati M, Ometto A, De Santolo A, Acciano S. Obstetric risk factors for periventricular leukomalacia among preterm infants. Obstet Gynaecol 1998;105:865–71. (Level II-2)

41. O'Shea TM, Kothadia JM, Roberst DD, Dillard RG. Perinatal events and the risk of intraparenchymal echodensity in very-low-birthweight neonates. Paediatr Perinat Epidemiol 1998;12:408–21. (Level II-2)

42. Murphy DJ, Sellers S, MacKenzie IZ, Yudkin PL, Johnson AM. Case-control study of antenatal and intrapartum risk factors for cerebral palsy in very preterm singleton babies. Lancet 1995;346:1449–54. (Level II-2)

43. Allan WC, Vohr B, Makuch RW, Katz KH, Ment LR. Antecedents of cerebral palsy in a multicenter trial of indomethacin for intraventricular hemorrhage. Arch Pediatr Adolesc Med 1997;151:580–5. (Level II-2)

44. Murphy DJ, Hope PL, Johnson A. Neonatal risk factors for cerebral palsy in very preterm babies: case-control study. BMJ 1997;314:404–8. (Level II-2)

45. Schrag SJ, Zywicki S, Farley MM, Reingold AL, Harrison LH, Lefkowitz LB, et al. Group B strepto-coccal disease in the era of intrapartum antibiotic prophylaxis. N Engl J Med 2000;342:15–20. (Level III)

46. Baker CJ. Group B streptococcal infection in newborns: prevention at last? [editorial] N Engl J Med 1986;314:1702–4. (Level III)

47. Klein JO. Bacterial sepsis and meningitis. In: Remington JS, Klein JO. Infectious diseases of the fetus and newborn infant. 5th ed. Philadelphia (PA): WB Saunders; 2001. p. 943–998. (Level III)

48. Mittendorf R, Covert R, Kohn J, Roizen N, Khoshnood B, Lee KS. The association of coagulase-negative staphylococci isolated from the chorioamnion at delivery and subsequent development of cerebral palsy. J Perinatol 2001;21:3–8. (Level II-2)

49. Wheeler AP, Bernard GR. Treating patients with severe sepsis. N Engl J Med 1999;340:207–14. (Level III)

50. Kraus FT, Acheen VI. Fetal thrombotic vasculopathy in the placenta: cerebral thrombi and infarcts, coagulopathies and cerebral palsy. Hum Pathol 1999;30: 759–69. (Level III)

51. Kraus FT. Cerebral palsy and thrombi in placental vessels of the fetus: insights from litigation. Hum Pathol 1997;28:246–8. (Level III)

52. Lockshin MD, Druzin ML, Goei S, Qamar T, Magid MS, Jovanovic L, et al. Antibody to cardiolipin as a predictor of fetal distress or death in pregnant patients with systemic lupus erythematosus. N Engl J Med 1985;313:152–6. (Level II-2)

53. Salafia CM, Parke AL. Placental pathology in systemic lupus erythematosus and phospholipid anitbody syndrome. Rheum Dis Clin North Am 1997; 23:85–97. (Level III)

54. Thorarensen O, Ryan S, Hunter J, Younkin DP. Factor V Leiden mutation: an unrecognized cause of hemiplegic cerebral palsy, neonatal stroke, and placental thrombosis. Ann Neurol 1997;42:372–5. (Level III)

55. Dizon-Townson DS, Meline L, Nelson LM, Varner M, Ward K. Fetal carriers of factor V Leiden mutation are prone to miscarriage and placental infarction. Am J Obstet Gynecol 1997;172:402–5. (Level II-2)

56. Lynch JK, Nelson KB, Curry CJ, Grether JK. Cerebrovascular disorders in children with the factor V Leiden mutation. J Child Neurol 2001;16:735–44. (Level III)

57. Reuss ML, Paneth N, Pinto-Martin JA, Lorenz JM, Susser M. The relation of transient hypothyroxinemia in preterm infants to neurologic development at two years of age. N Engl J Med 1996;334:821–7. (Level II-2)

58. Lucas A, Rennie J, Baker BA, Morley R. Low plasma triiodothyronine concentrations and outcome in preterm infants. Arch Dis Child 1988;631:1201–6. (Level II-2)

59. Meijer WJ, Verloove-Vanhorick SP, Brand R, van den Brande JL. Transient hypothyroxinemia associated

with developmental delay in very preterm infants. Arch Dis Child 1992;67:944–7. (Level II-2)

60. Den Ouden AL, Kok JH, Verkerk PH, Brand R, Verloove-Vanhorick SP. The relation between neonatal thyroxine levels and neurodevelopmental outcome at age 5 and 9 years in a national cohort of very preterm and/or very low birth weight infants. Pediatr Res 1996;39:142–5. (Level II-2)

61. Osborn DA. Thyroid hormones for preventing neurodevelopmental impairment in preterm infants (Cochrane Review). In: The Cochrane Library, Issue 4, 2001. Oxford: Update Software. (Meta-analysis)

62. Badawi N, Kurinczuk JJ, Mackenzie CL, Keogh JM, Burton PR, Pemberton PJ, et al. Maternal thyroid disease: a risk factor for newborn encephalopathy in term infants. BJOG 2000;107:798–801. (Level III)

63. Nelson KB, Ellenberg JH. Antecedents of cerebral palsy. I Univariate analysis of risks. Am J Dis Child 1985;139:1031–8. (Level II-2)

64. Nelson KB, Ellenberg JH. Antecedents of cerebral palsy. Multivariate analysis of risk. N Engl J Med 1986;315:81–6. (Level II-2)

65. Stanley F, Blair E, Alberman E. Causal pathways in initiated preconceptionally or in early pregnancy. In: Cerebral palsies: epidemiology and causal pathways. London: Mac Keith Press; 2000. p. 48–59. (Level III)

66. Castoldi AF, Coccini T, Ceccatelli S, Manzo L. Neurotoxicity and molecular effects of methylmercury. Brain Res Bull 2001;55:197–203. (Level III)

67. Brodsky JB, Cohen EN, Whitcher C, Brown BW Jr, Wu ML. Occupational exposure to mercury in denistry and pregnancy outcome. J Am Dent Assoc 1985:111:779–80. (Level II-3)

68. Ericson A, Kallen B. Pregnancy outcome in women working as dentists, dental assistants, or dental technicians. Int Arch Occup Environ Health 1989;61: 329–33. (Level III)

69. Needleman HL, Rabinowitz M, Leviton A, Linn S, Schoenbaum S. The relationships between prenatal exposure to lead and congenital anomalies. JAMA 1981;251:2956–9. (Level II-3)

70. Wigg NR, Vimpani GV, McMichael AJ, Baghurst PA, Robertson EF, Roberts RJ. Port Pirie Cohort study: childhood blood lead and neuropsychological development at age two years. J Epimedmiol Community Health 1988;42:213–9. (Level II-3)

71. McMichael AJ, Vimpani GV, Robertson EF, Baghurst PA, Clark PD. The Port Pirie cohort study: maternal blood lead and pregnancy outcome. J Epidemiol Community Health 1986;40:18–25. (Level II-2)

72. Milunsky A, Ulcickas M, Rothman KJ, Willett W, Jick SS, Jick H. Maternal heat exposure and neural tube defects. JAMA 1992;268:882–5. (Level II-2)

73. McDonald JC, Lavoie J, Cote R, McDonald AD. Chemical exposures at work in early pregnancy and congenital defect: a case-referent study. Br J Ind Med 1987;44:527 33. (Level II 2)

74. Jones KL, Smith DW, Ulleland CN, Streissguth AP. Pattern of malformation in offspring of chronic alcoholic mothers. Lancet 1973;1:1267–71. (Level III)

75. Abel EL. An update on incidence of FAS: FAS is not an equal opportunity birth defect. Neurotoxicol Teratol 1995;17:437–43. (Level III)

76. Streissguth AP, Clarren SK, Jones KL. Natural history of the fetal alcohol syndrome: a 10-year follow-up of eleven patients. Lancet 1985;2(8446):85–91. (Level III)

77. American Academy of Pediatrics. Committee on Substance Abuse and Committee on Children with Disabilities. Fetal alcohol syndrome and alcohol-related neurodevelopmental disorders. Pediatrics 2000; 106:358–61. (Level III)

78. Chasnoff IJ, Bussey ME, Savich R, Stack CM. Perinatal cerebral infarction and maternal cocaine use. J Pediatr 1986;108:456–9. (Level III)

79. Kapur RP, Shaw CM, Shepard TH. Brain hemorrhages in cocaine-exposed human fetuses. Teratology 1991:44:11–8. (Level III)

80. Smit BJ, Bor K, Van Huis AM, Lie A, Ling IS, Schmidt SC. Cocaine use in Amsterdam. Acta Pediatr Suppl 1994:32–5. (Level III)

81. Telsey AM, Merrit TA, Dixon SD. Cocaine exposure in a term neonate. Necrotizing enterocolitis as a complication. Clin Pediatr 1988;27:547–50. (Level III)

82. Tenorio GM, Nazvi M, Bickers GH, Hubbird RH. Intrauterine stroke and maternal polydrug abuse. Case report. Clin Pediatr 1988;27:565–7. (Level III)

83. van de Bor M, Walther FJ, Sims ME. Increased cerebral blood flow velocity in infants of mothers who abuse cocaine. Pediatrics 1990;85:733–6. (Level II-2)

84. Eyler FD, Behnke M, Conlon M, Woods NS, Wobie K. Birth outcome from a prospective, matched study of prenatal crack/cocaine use: I. Interactive and dose effects on health and growth. Pediatrics 1998;101: 229–37. (Level II-2)

85. Bateman DA, Chiriboga CA. Dose-response effect of cocaine on newborn head circumference. Pediatrics 2000;106:E33. Available at http://www.pediatrics.org/. Retrieved November 30, 2001 (Level II-2)

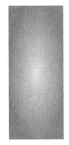

CHAPTER 3

ANTEPARTUM AND INTRAPARTUM CONSIDERATIONS AND ASSESSMENT

Antepartum Events

Most cases of cerebral palsy are related to antepartum factors and not to isolated intrapartum events or difficulties during the labor or delivery process. Antepartum conditions associated with cerebral palsy include preterm birth; intrauterine infections, such as chorioamnionitis; intrauterine growth restriction; multiple pregnancies; coagulation disorders; antepartum bleeding; congenital or genetic anomalies; and infertility treatment.

Preconceptional and antepartum risk factors are different for neonatal encephalopathy than for cerebral palsy. Although these conditions are often considered together, it is important to distinguish them. Infants with cerebral palsy frequently do not have neonatal encephalopathy, which implies the two conditions may represent different types of and time intervals for cerebral damage. Risk factors for neonatal encephalopathy are increasing maternal age, family history of neurologic disorders, maternal thyroid disease, maternal hypertension, vaginal bleeding, infertility, and evidence of growth restriction (1).

Evaluation of data from the National Collaborative Perinatal Project for antepartum events demonstrated various complications associated with an increase in cerebral palsy rates, but the absolute rates observed for each specific condition were not high, and none were more than 2% in babies weighing more than 2,500 g at birth. The complications as related to cerebral palsy became important when the 5-minute Apgar score was between 0 and 3 for the conditions of polyhydramnios, decreased fetal heart rate (<100 beats per minute), and nuchal cord. There was no increase in the risk of cerebral palsy following an obstetric complication if the 5-minute Apgar score was 7 or greater (2). Univariate analysis of these data revealed that a maternal history of mental retardation, seizures, hyperthyroidism, or unusual or long menstrual cycles was associated with an increased risk of cerebral palsy (3). In infants weighing more than 2,500 g at birth, maternal seizures, severe proteinuria, third-trimester bleeding, and polyhydramnios were statistically significant indicators for risk of cerebral palsy (3). A multivariate analysis of the same data revealed that the 95% confidence intervals for these variables all crossed one, thus failing to achieve statistical significance (4). Evaluation of the California Child Health and Development Study demonstrated that long menstrual cycles (>36 days), polyhydramnios, and unusual pregnancy intervals (<3 months or >3 years) to be statistically significant with 95% confidence intervals that did not cross one (5). Specific gestational age data were not given.

A multivariate analysis of 164 cases and 400 controls evaluated the role of preconceptional, antepartum, and intrapartum factors in neonatal encephalopathy (1). The strongest antepartum risk factor for neonatal encephalopathy was fetal growth restriction. There are, however, many different causes of fetal growth restriction, and each may differ in its capacity to cause or predispose a fetus to neonatal encephalopathy. The risk for neonatal encephalopathy also increased with each advancing week of gestation after 38 weeks. Several sociodemographic characteristics were significant risk factors for neonatal encephalopathy. Maternal seizures, maternal thyroid disease, bleeding in pregnancy, an excess of congenital anomalies, and markers of prenatal and perinatal infection were also associated with neonatal encephalopathy, supporting the idea of multiple causal pathways leading to neonatal encephalopathy and cerebral palsy (1). Of significance, however, was that 70% of cases of neonatal encephalopathy were probably caused by events arising before the onset of labor. Infants with neonatal encephalopathy experienced a more adverse antepartum course than controls, and intrapartum hypoxia less frequently was the sole cause of neonatal encephalopathy.

Conclusions

- There are numerous periconceptional and antenatal antecedents for both neonatal encephalopathy and cerebral palsy.

- Most known conditions associated with either neonatal encephalopathy or cerebral palsy are related to abnormal antepartum conditions rarely amenable to intervention by the health care provider.

Fetal Heart Rate Monitoring

Physiologic Basis

Alterations in blood flow and oxygen content of the maternal, uteroplacental, or umbilical circulations can result in fetal hypoxia. Certain fetal heart rate patterns indicate possible mechanisms for decreased fetal oxygenation.

Uteroplacental insufficiency can result if the maternal blood flow or blood oxygen content are diminished. Uterine contractions produce intermittent diminution of blood flow to the intervillous space where oxygen exchange occurs (6). If this intermittent interruption of flow exceeds a critical level, the fetal heart rate responds specifically with a pattern of late deceleration. Late deceleration begins as a vagal reflex; when fetal oxygenation is sufficiently impaired to produce fetal metabolic acidosis from anaerobic glycolysis, direct myocardial depression occurs (7). When the late deceleration is of the reflex type, the fetal heart rate tracing characteristically has good variability and fetal reactivity, but as the fetus develops metabolic acidosis, the fetal heart rate loses its variability. When the fetal pH is less than 7.20, the fetal heart rate reactivity, either spontaneous or evoked, may disappear (8, 9). If uteroplacental oxygen transfer is acutely and substantially impaired, the resulting fetal heart rate pattern is a prolonged deceleration. Clinical events associated with acute uteroplacental insufficiency are uterine rupture, maternal cardiovascular collapse, total placental abruption, and tetanic uterine contractions. Similarly, with total cord occlusion, a prolonged deceleration will develop.

When the umbilical cord is compressed, a fetal heart rate pattern of variable deceleration develops (10). This is characterized by rapid onset and resolution and bears no specific relation to the time during contractions that the deceleration begins. Usually, the cord compression is mild and of no consequence. There may be a transient elevation of the fetal P_{CO_2} (partial pressure of carbon dioxide), but significant hypoxia usually does not develop. If cord compression is prolonged, significant fetal hypoxia can occur. When this happens, the return to baseline becomes gradual, the duration of the deceleration may increase, and frequently, the fetal heart rate variability will decrease and the baseline fetal heart rate may increase.

Antepartum Fetal Monitoring and Neonatal Encephalopathy

Because of the difficulties with long-term follow up, very few studies have looked at the relationship between antepartum fetal testing and long-term neurologic outcome. Several randomized prospective trials using weekly nonstress test surveillance have shown no benefit (11–14). The rest of the literature on nonstress tests involves nonrandomized, usually retrospective reviews. The only prospective, randomized trial of antepartum fetal evaluation that showed benefit involved instructing women in fetal movement counts and showed a decreased occurrence of fetal death but no impact on long-term neurologic outcomes (15).

In 1983, an Australian study showed that among 72 patients with a nonreactive positive spontaneous contraction stress test result, there was a 28% perinatal mortality rate; of the 52 infants that survived the neonatal period, 45 were assessed and 27% were found to have a neurologic handicap (16). A retrospective study using biophysical profile as the primary means of surveillance reported the incidence of cerebral palsy was 1.33 per 1,000 in the group with biophysical profile and 4.74 per 1,000 in those patients not monitored with biophysical profile testing (17).

There is evidence that abnormal test results are found more frequently in patients with abnormal neurologic outcome. However, the predictive value of antenatal testing remains poor because of the high frequency of abnormal test results in patients with normal outcome.

Intrapartum Fetal Monitoring and Neonatal Encephalopathy

Before the 1970s, the only widely available clinical techniques used to evaluate the intrapartum condition of the fetus were the appearance of amniotic fluid and auscultated fetal bradycardia. An analysis of the National Collaborative Perinatal Project data concluded auscultatory fetal heart rate monitoring was of little value (18). With the advent of intrapartum electronic fetal heart rate monitoring, a number of early nonrandomized, mainly historically controlled and mostly retrospective studies suggested a benefit to intrapartum fetal heart rate monitoring, primarily for high-risk patients (19–26). Many believed intrapartum fetal heart rate monitoring would prove beneficial in decreasing the incidence of cerebral palsy and mental retardation (27). Specifically, there were fewer cases of intrapartum and neonatal death in patients who had intrapartum fetal heart rate monitoring, and some studies showed fewer low Apgar scores, as well as less need for resuscitation.

In the late 1970s and early 1980s, a number of prospectively randomized trials compared intrapartum fetal heart rate monitoring with careful auscultation, usually with one-on-one nursing. These trials failed to show any benefit of electronic fetal monitoring with respect to fetal or neonatal death, Apgar scores, fetal pH, need for resuscitation, or neonatal intensive care unit admissions (28-33). Some studies showed increased cesarean delivery rates in patients who had intrapartum electronic fetal heart rate monitoring, which led to criticism of fetal heart rate monitoring from a cost–benefit standpoint and controversy over the value of the technique (34, 35).

The only benefit seen for intrapartum fetal heart rate monitoring in the randomized trials was a decreased incidence of neonatal seizures in the Dublin trial (36). When all the studies were subjected to a meta-analysis, it appeared neonatal seizures were indeed fewer among patients who had intrapartum fetal heart rate monitoring (37, 38). Long-term follow-up studies, however, failed to show any decrease in abnormal neurologic outcome between those who had electronic monitoring and those who did not (37). No prospective randomized trials have compared either intrapartum fetal heart rate monitoring or intermittent auscultation with no monitoring.

The correlation of intrapartum fetal heart rate patterns with outcome is problematic. Even if intrapartum fetal heart rate patterns were predictive of all bad outcome from hypoxia, there would be no value unless the patterns gave sufficient warning to allow the clinician to intervene and take appropriate action to prevent the bad outcome. If, however, abnormal patterns did give warning in sufficient time to prevent a bad outcome, there would be no correlation with outcome. Fetuses who are severely asphyxiated during the intrapartum period will have abnormal fetal heart rate patterns (39). However, most patients with nonreassuring fetal heart rate patterns give birth to neonates with normal Apgar scores (40). Abnormal electronic fetal heart patterns are poor predictors of subsequent development of cerebral palsy (41).

The use of fetal scalp blood sampling for patients with nonreassuring patterns has been shown to be associated with decreased need for operative intervention (29). However, fetal scalp blood sampling use has decreased as fetal scalp stimulation and vibroacoustic stimulation have proved to be easier ways to assure a normal fetal pH when evoked accelerations occur (8, 42).

The U.S. Food and Drug Administration has approved labeling for the use of fetal pulse oximetry for patients with nonreassuring fetal heart rate patterns. A large randomized clinical trial of fetal pulse oximetry showed a decrease in cesarean delivery for nonreassuring fetal heart rate patterns but a corresponding increase in cesarean delivery for dystocia. Neonatal outcomes were similar in the fetal pulse oximetry group when compared with a group with nonreassuring patterns managed without fetal pulse oximetry (43). Further studies are needed before this technique can be considered standard practice.

The incidence of cerebral palsy has remained essentially unchanged despite the common use of intrapartum fetal heart rate monitoring in both high- and low-risk patients. This should not be surprising inasmuch as previous beliefs regarding the dominant contribution of intrapartum hypoxia to subsequent neurologic abnormalities are unfounded (44–46).

Current Role of Intrapartum Electronic Fetal Heart Rate Monitoring

Before randomized controlled trials, 135,000 patients in nonrandomized trials of either continuous electronic monitoring or nonintensive fetal monitoring by auscultation were compared. The intrapartum fetal death rate in the electronically monitored group was 0.54 per 1,000 compared with 1.76 per 1,000 in the nonintensively auscultated group. This resulted in a fetal death ratio of 3.26, favoring electronic intrapartum fetal monitoring ($P = <0.05$) (47). In randomized controlled trials comparing electronic monitoring to intermittent auscultation, the auscultation group had an intensive protocol that consisted of a one-on-one nurse listening every 15 minutes in the first stage of labor and every 5 minutes in the second stage of labor. The intrapartum fetal death rate in both groups was comparable to the intrapartum fetal death rate in the nonrandomized electronically monitored group (28–31). Thus, it would appear that intensive intrapartum fetal monitoring by either auscultation or continuous electronic monitoring is better than nonintensive auscultation for the prevention of intrapartum fetal death. Although the use of fetal heart rate monitoring has led to a decrease in intrapartum fetal deaths, the incidence of cerebral palsy has not changed since its introduction.

The specific issue of the value of electronic fetal monitoring as a predictor of cerebral palsy has been addressed (41). No association has been determined between the highest or lowest fetal heart rate and the risk of cerebral palsy. The two findings associated with the development of cerebral palsy were repetitive late decelerations of the fetal heart rate and a decrease in beat-to-beat variability. These findings were uncommon in infants weighing more than 2,500 g. Also, these monitor findings had a very high false-positive rate for predicting cerebral palsy.

The National Institute of Child Health and Human Development consensus report stated a normal fetal heart tracing consisting of a normal baseline rate, moderate fetal heart rate variability, presence of accelerations, and absence of decelerations is extremely predictive of a normally oxygenated fetus. The report also said patterns predictive of current or impending asphyxia placing the fetus at risk for neurologic damage include recurrent late or severe variable decelerations or substantial bradycardia, with absent fetal heart rate variability.

For intrapartum asphyxia to develop in a fetus that was previously normal at the start of labor, some major, or sentinel event must occur. If the fetus is undergoing continuous electronic fetal heart rate monitoring, the sentinel event should result in either an abnormal tracing with either a prolonged deceleration, repetitive late decelerations, and/or repetitive severe variable decelerations and decreased fetal heart rate variability. In the circumstance of a woman who presents in labor with an abnormal fetal heart rate that was present for an unknown period, and demonstrating one or all of the previous patterns, the fetus may have already experienced damage and rapid delivery may not improve the outcome.

Conclusions

- Specific fetal heart rate patterns are associated with uteroplacental insufficiency and umbilical cord compression. Acute profound hypoxia from any cause results in a prolonged deceleration. Neonatal encephalopathy may result from severe fetal hypoxia from any cause.

- No randomized controlled trials have shown that any form of antenatal testing will decrease the incidence of cerebral palsy.

- Fetal movement counting may decrease antenatal death rates.

- Intrapartum electronic fetal heart rate monitoring is associated with fewer cases of neonatal seizures than dedicated fetal heart rate auscultation.

- Intrapartum fetal heart rate monitoring is not associated with a decrease in cerebral palsy when compared with patients with dedicated fetal heart auscultation.

- Abnormal fetal heart patterns have an extraordinarily high false-positive rate of predicting the development of cerebral palsy.

Neonatal Neurologic Outcome Following Acute Catastrophic Intrapartum Asphyxia: The Effect of Time from Diagnosis to Delivery

Animal data show that the duration and degree of fetal hypoxia are related to the occurrence and extent of brain damage. The data in humans, however, are not as clear because the situation in humans does not allow experimental manipulation to determine the different factors involved. In humans, information is extrapolated from actual cases of umbilical cord prolapse, abruptio placenta, shoulder dystocia, maternal cardiac arrest, and catastrophic uterine rupture. A multitude of clinical factors surrounding these conditions affect the neurologic outcome of the fetus. Included are the degree and duration of cord compression (complete versus variable), the degree and duration of placental separation, the effectiveness and duration of maternal cardiopulmonary resuscitation, and the fetal condition before the event (a normal fetus versus one compromised by preexisting uteroplacental insufficiency or intermittent cord occlusion). Fetal outcome also will likely be affected by the length of time between actual occurrence of the event, diagnosis, and the ability to effect termination of the insult.

The pattern of neurologic injury following acute catastrophic hypoxic–ischemic insult can involve the thalami and basal ganglia predominantly and may be different from the common pattern following chronic insult in the term newborn that involves predominantly the cerebral cortex and the subcortical white matter (48, 49). This pattern was found to be highly predictive of poor outcome and corresponds closely to experimental models of acute total perinatal asphyxia (50). In a review of infants hospitalized in an infant special care unit, 85 developed neonatal seizures. Eleven of those infants had a gestational age beyond 37 weeks at delivery and had experienced persistent prolonged decelerations without recovery just before delivery (49). Radiologic and clinical findings showed a consistent pattern of injury in the subcortical brain nuclei with complete or relative sparing of the cerebral cortex and white matter, along with absent or only subtle injury to organs other than the brain.

As noted, fetal asphyxial brain injury secondary to acute catastrophic intrapartum events may not be associated with other multiorgan system injury (49, 51). In a review of 14 cases of severe fetal brain injury with absent multiorgan system dysfunction associated with acute intrapartum asphyxial events (six uterine ruptures, five prolonged fetal heart rate decelerations, one fetal exsanguination, one umbilical cord prolapse, and one maternal cardiopulmonary arrest), the average duration of the prolonged fetal heart rate deceleration was 32.1 ± 9.1 minutes (range: 19–51 minutes) (51). The higher metabolic rate of subcortical nuclei compared with the cerebral hemispheres and of the brain compared with other organs may explain the distribution of cerebral damage and yet the sparing of other organs that can be seen with an abrupt decrease in oxygenation following acute near-total asphyxia. Alternatively, the shunting of blood flow from other organs to the brain and from the cerebral hemispheres to the thalamus and brainstem may explain the involvement of the cerebral hemispheres and multiorgan dysfunction seen with the more prolonged type of fetal hypoxia associated with uteroplacental ischemia. Finally, the pattern of the hypoxic–ischemic insult (chronic versus acute), the gestational age of the fetus, and the effectiveness of resuscitation all will have bearing on the ultimate neurologic outcome. For example, in sheep, complete umbilical cord occlusion of up to 20 minutes did not result in neurologic damage in mid gestation (52), while repeated brief umbilical cord occlusions in near-term fetal lambs did result in neurologic damage (53). The lower level of cerebral metabolism in early gestation compared with term gestation and the more cytotoxic effects of the ischemia-reperfusion insult compared with continuous ischemia may explain these differences.

Nonhuman Primate Models of Asphyxia

The oxygen content of blood in the abdominal aorta of the fetal monkey at term can decrease through a wide range before any changes are observed in vital signs or central nervous system function (mild asphyxia starting at partial pressure of oxygen of 28–30 mm Hg, hemoglobin saturation of 60–70%, and oxygen content of 10–12 vol % (54). Fetal vital signs start to change as the arterial oxygen content decreases into the moderate asphyxia range (moderate asphyxia starting at partial pressure of oxygen of 15–16 mm Hg, hemoglobin saturation of 25–30%, and oxygen content of 3–4 vol %). Fetal oxygenation can remain in this range for prolonged periods (beyond 1–2 hours) without producing brain injury or other abnormalities. However, evidence of brain damage occurs regularly when levels of severe asphyxia are maintained beyond 10–15 minutes (severe asphyxia starting at partial pressure of oxygen of 11–12 mm Hg, hemoglobin saturation of 12–14%, and oxygen content of 0.8–1.5 vol %).

A different experimental model that more closely resembles acute catastrophic events, such as cord prolapse or uterine rupture, evaluated the effect of acute total perinatal asphyxia on brain pathology in term monkey fetuses (55). Acute total asphyxia was produced by clamping the umbilical cord and slipping a thin, saline-filled, rubber sac over the fetal head at surgical delivery. The envelopment of the fetal head prevented the onset of air breathing for a specified period, following which resuscitation was performed. The first evidence of brain damage in survivors occurred at 10 minutes of total asphyxia. Fetuses asphyxiated for longer than 25 minutes died in the early hours in the intensive care unit from myocardial injury. The ranking of brain structures in order of susceptibility to injury correlated with their volume flow of blood per unit of time under normal conditions; a direct reflection of their metabolic rate. Substantial differences in the distribution of cerebral pathology exist between acute total asphyxia and episodic, prolonged partial asphyxia. It should be emphasized that the outcome of these animals depended on the resuscitation efforts, and the same is probably true for the human neonate as well. This review was mostly descriptive and contained very little data. Studies by these and other authors also suggest the pathologic consequences of asphyxia are gestational-age dependent, with the mid-gestation monkey fetus withstanding up to 30 minutes of cord clamping without sustaining detectable pathology, whereas only 10 minutes in the term fetus are sufficient to produce serious damage (56, 57). Again, the data from these investigations were limited or unavailable for review.

In addition to blood oxygen content, tissue perfusion is critical to the development of neurologic damage. The combination of hypoxia and hypotension was more detrimental to cerebral metabolism of mid-gestation sheep fetuses than hypoxia alone (58). Fetal hypotension or hypovolemia or both, which occur frequently in conditions associated with acute catastrophic asphyxia such as uterine rupture and abruptio placenta, may be as important a determinant of neurologic outcome as hypoxemia.

The limitations of animal models for the study of perinatal hypoxic–ischemic encephalopathy are well recognized: they include standardization of experimental design and applicability to the human infant (59). Perhaps even more importantly, in most of the animal models used the fetus or neonate is far more advanced neurologically than the human counterpart at every gestational age.

It also is important to emphasize that most of the information on animal models published in the 1960s, 1970s, and the early 1980s is in the form of reviews that omit important details such as number of animals, methods, and data. These deficiencies limit our ability to reproduce these experiments and, more importantly, to objectively evaluate the soundness of the conclusions or opinions (55, 60). Investigators also have concluded, "The brainstem injury pattern produced in the monkey fetus by total asphyxia bears no relation to the brain pathology typifying human perinatal damage" (55). Others have said, "The validity of findings in the nonhuman primate models also need to be established using advanced neurological methods, since there are considerable differences between the status of the neonatal brain in humans and in monkeys and apes..." (59). They also note, "At birth the human brain is immature relative to that of the

newborn baboon and chimpanzee," and "Unlike any other mammal, the human nervous system has the greatest potential for postnatal growth and maturation" (59). Advances in neuroimaging techniques and other diagnostic modalities argue strongly for repeating some of the experiments in these animal models.

Fetal Oxygenation and Acid–Base Parameters in Humans

It is difficult to determine how the thresholds for oxygenation parameters in the nonhuman primate compare with those in the human fetus, because corresponding data from human fetuses in utero are scarce. The closest values to the fetal condition in utero may be those obtained by cordocentesis. A number of studies have reported on these values (61–65). In practically all cases, the cordocentesis was not elective and was performed for a number of different clinical indications.

The data for normal values were obtained from those fetuses who were either unaffected by the condition under investigation or whose condition was one which was deemed to not affect blood gas and acid–base status. Gestational ages ranged from the early second trimester until term, and blood gas values varied significantly with advancing gestation. Because of the nature of the indication, the number of cases at term was limited. In most cases, the umbilical venous blood was sampled. The results, therefore, reflected placental blood gas exchange rather than fetal status. In two reports that included analysis of umbilical arterial blood, the sampling was performed fetoscopically in heavily sedated mothers, possibly affecting the results (62, 63). Judging by the similarities between these two reports, the same cases may have been included twice.

In one of the largest studies, blood gas and acid–base status were evaluated in umbilical artery blood obtained by cordocentesis without sedation in 35 appropriate-growth-for-gestational-age fetuses (mean gestational age: 25 weeks) deemed to have normal oxygenation. Reference ranges for pH, Po_2, and Pco_2 versus gestational age were constructed using least-square analysis.

Unfortunately, these reference ranges were only given graphically. From these graphs, the mean (95% confidence interval) values at 38 weeks appear to be in the vicinity of 7.35 (7.29–7.41) for pH, 23 (14–32) mm Hg for P_{O_2}, and 42 (38–46) mm Hg for P_{CO_2} (61).

Although analysis of umbilical blood obtained at cordocentesis may approximate fetal condition more closely than analysis of cord blood obtained immediately following uncomplicated elective cesarean delivery in the absence of labor, the latter method has provided more data from cases at term. Mean ± standard deviation for umbilical artery pH, P_{CO_2}, and base excess in 26 uncomplicated cases undergoing elective cesarean delivery before labor were 7.32 ± 0.06, 44.2 ± 9 mm Hg, and –2.3 ± 3.9 mmol/L, respectively. In the group who had elective cesarean delivery before labor, the pH was higher, the P_{CO_2} was lower, and the base excess was higher than in the groups delivered vaginally or by cesarean delivery during labor (66). In a different study, percent oxygen saturation calculated from umbilical artery P_{O_2} and pH in 665 cases delivered by elective cesarean delivery (presumably uncomplicated cases delivered at term and before labor) was 23 ± 14% and was higher than found in cases delivered by cesarean after labor (18 ± 13%; n = 1,609) but not different than the vaginal delivery group (24 ± 15%; n = 14,285) (67).

Umbilical Cord Prolapse

Fetal hypoxia in umbilical cord prolapse is the result of impediment to blood flow to and from the placenta. This occlusion may or may not be continuous or complete. Thus, one would postulate that injury patterns might resemble acute total fetal asphyxia, acute partial intermittent asphyxia, or a hybrid of the two. The relationship between time-to-delivery and neurologic outcome in cord prolapse depends on fetal presentation, station, and the frequency of contractions in addition to the other factors affecting neurologic outcome listed previously. Cord compression in cephalic presentation would generally be more severe than in a transverse lie.

Most of the data regarding neonatal outcome following cord prolapse dates back 20 or more years and may have limited applicability today. Historic differences in fetal heart rate monitoring practice, choice of delivery method (vaginal versus cesarean delivery, especially for breech presentation), neonatal resuscitation, and the changing threshold for both viability of preterm neonates as well as gestational-age-specific long-term morbidity all affect fetal outcome. Because the variables are so great, only the following broad generalizations can be made, and even then exceptions will be common.

- Fetal mortality is affected by the time from diagnosis to delivery (68).

- Perinatal mortality is greatest with frank prolapse, followed by occult prolapse, and least in controls without prolapse (69, 70).

- By far the most common long-term neurologic outcome with either frank or occult cord prolapse is a normal infant (69–71).

Shoulder Dystocia

The issues with shoulder dystocia are similar to those of cord prolapse, with the exception that the degree of umbilical cord compression can usually be assumed to be at least as severe or more severe than seen with umbilical cord prolapse. The same generalizations regarding outcome can again be assumed.

In a review of 56 cases of fatal shoulder dystocia, the head-to-body delivery interval was recorded by the clinical staff involved as less than 5 minutes in 47% of cases and greater than 10 minutes in 20% of cases (72). The authors determined nonreassuring fetal status ("fetal distress") was present in 14 cases before delivery of the head. The incidence of fetal compromise during labor was not different between neonates who died following a short versus long head-to-body delivery interval. Thirty-eight (68%) newborns had no signs of life at delivery, and 23 of these could not be resuscitated and were classified as stillborn. Twenty-one neonates were transferred to a neonatal unit, most with major postnatal complications such as hypoxic–ischemic encephalopathy. Adequate autopsies were performed on 18 cases, with evidence of acute hypoxic organ damage in 96% of cases and birth trauma in 24%. Unfortunately, details regarding the site and type of organ injury were not provided.

Uterine Rupture

In addition to the numerous maternal and fetal factors listed previously, perinatal mortality and morbidity with uterine rupture is greatly affected by whether the fetus was extruded from the uterus. One review of all cases of uterine rupture, defined as symptomatic uterine scar separation that required emergency laparotomy, identified 106 cases out of 11,179 women with a previous cesarean delivery who underwent trial of labor (73). Of the 99 cases with complete maternal and neonatal records, the fetuses were totally extruded in 28, partially extruded in 13, and not extruded in 58. The number of fetuses with perinatal death, cases of perinatal asphyxia (defined as an umbilical artery pH <7 with seizures and multiorgan dysfunction), need for ventilatory support, 5-minute Apgar score less than 7, and umbilical artery pH less than 7 were all much worse with total or partial fetal extrusion from the uterine cavity than when the fetus remained in utero, as would be expected.

The authors did not comment on the neurologic outcome of the neonates or specifically analyze the relationship between neurologic outcome and the time from diagnosis to delivery, but some of the data provided may be useful in this regard. Four of the perinatal deaths (3 of the 4 deaths with total extrusion and 1 of 2 deaths in the nonextrusion group) occurred in 13 women who had nonreassuring fetal status ("acute fetal distress") on admission and who underwent immediate cesarean delivery. In these cases, fetal damage may well have occurred before presentation, and the duration of the insult cannot be determined. Of the remaining nine cases, three had an umbilical artery pH less than 7.

The implications are that the insult may have occurred long before admission and that intrapartum management could not have prevented the outcome. Fetal heart rate patterns were analyzed for abnormalities on the remaining cases after excluding the 13 patients who were delivered immediately and the eight patients who were delivered vaginally without nonreassuring fetal status. Prolonged decelerations that provoked operative delivery occurred in 55 of the remaining 78 women (see Fig. 3–1). No significant perinatal morbidity occurred in patients whose only fetal heart rate abnormality was prolonged deceleration when delivery occurred within 17 minutes of the onset of the prolonged deceleration.

Perinatal asphyxia occurred as early as 10 minutes after the onset of prolonged deceleration when the prolonged deceleration was preceded by a period of severe late decelerations ranging from 36 to 90 minutes in duration. There was significant overlap in the time from onset of prolonged deceleration to delivery between cases with perinatal morbidity and those without complications, regardless of the presence or absence of antecedent fetal heart rate abnormalities. The time from the onset of the prolonged deceleration to delivery was 13 ± 6.5 minutes in the neonates without significant morbidity.

A retrospective study identified 11 women who had intrapartum uterine rupture among 3,353 women who attempted vaginal birth after previous cesarean delivery between 1990 and 1995 (74). Nine of the 11 women (73%) had fetal heart rate bradycardia before delivery, all lasting longer than 15 minutes, with five episodes lasting between 18 and 37 minutes. Before the bradycardia, four had late decelerations, eight had variable decelerations, and three had early decelerations. All but one of the neonates had a cord blood pH less than 7, and five had a base excess greater than 15 mEq/L (not specified arterial or venous). The author noted a trend toward lower pH and higher base excess that appeared to be related to the length of the bradycardia but did not provide the data. Eight of the 11 neonates were admitted to the neonatal intensive care unit, but only one required hospitalization beyond age 5 days. None of the neonates had seizures or multiorgan dysfunction, and none required ventilatory assistance. One neonate was referred to the neurologic clinic but was lost to follow-up. None of the neonates had sustained brain damage as of the time of publication.

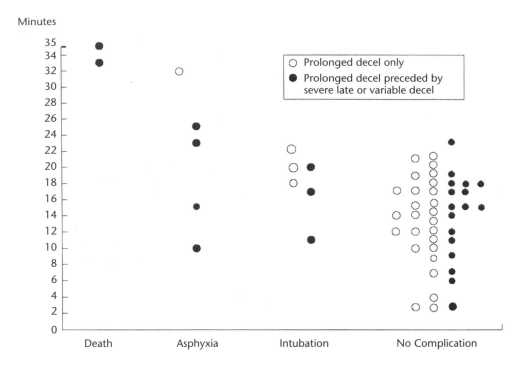

Fig. 3.1. Immediate neonatal outcome in cases of uterine rupture relative to fetal heart rate pattern and interval to delivery. (Leung AS, Leung EK, Paul RH. Uterine rupture after previous cesarean delivery: maternal and fetal consequences. Am J Obstet Gynecol 1993;169:945–50.)

Maternal Cardiopulmonary Arrest

A number of case studies have attempted to report on the relationship between the interval from cardiopulmonary arrest to delivery and neonatal outcome. As with other acute catastrophic causes of fetal asphyxia, neonatal outcome following cardiopulmonary arrest depends on a number of factors that may be independent of the duration zof the asphyxial episode, including the cause of cardiopulmonary arrest (eg, trauma, amniotic fluid embolism, medical complications), the maternal status and maternal stability or instability before the arrest, the efficacy of cardiopulmonary resuscitation, and the gestational age of the fetus (preterm birth may occur in trauma cases).

One report on neonatal outcomes in women with amniotic fluid embolism included in a national registry identified 69 cases, of which 25 met strict inclusion criteria and had cardiac arrest while the fetus was alive in utero (75). The precise arrest-to-delivery time was available in 16

of the 25 women. Neurologically intact survival was inversely related to the time from cardiac arrest to delivery. The limitations of these data include reporting bias, unknown criteria for ascertainment of outcome, and lack of information regarding associated obstetric conditions (eg, abruptio placenta, uterine rupture), maternal status before cardiac arrest, or efficacy of cardiovascular resuscitation.

A review of the topic summarized the data published from 1900 to 1985 regarding neonatal outcome in relation to the time from maternal death to delivery (76). The authors noted that most fetal survivors were delivered within 5 minutes, and only rare healthy survivors were reported among fetuses delivered more than 10 minutes after cardiopulmonary arrest (Table 3–1). The limitations of these data include reporting bias, unknown criteria for ascertainment of outcome, and unclear number of postmortem cesarean deliveries performed for nonsurviving infants.

Table 3–1. Postmortem Cesarean Deliveries with Surviving Infants According to Time from Death of the Mother Until Delivery

Time (min)	No. Cases, Outcome	Percentage of Total
0–5	12 normal infants	70
6–10	7 normal, 1 mild neurologic sequelae	13
11–15	6 normal, 1 severe neurologic sequelae	12
16–20	1 severe neurologic sequelae	1.7
≥21	1 normal, 2 severe neurologic sequelae	3.3

Katz VL, Dotters DJ, Droegemueller W. Perimortem cesarean delivery. Obstet Gynecol 1986;68:571–6.

Survival of an infant delivered 22 minutes after medically documented maternal cardiac arrest has been reported (77). At age 18 months, the child was clinically normal except for persistent mild hypotonia, and her Denver Developmental Screening Test Scores were normal.

The "30-Minute Rule"

There has been much controversy regarding the so-called "30-minute rule"—the capability to begin a cesarean delivery within 30 minutes of the decision to perform it (78). This arbitrary time limit was implemented to encourage hospitals with obstetric services to provide anesthetic resources and operating rooms, as well as nursing, obstetric, and pediatric personnel who can perform cesarean delivery and neonatal resuscitation in a timely fashion. Cesarean delivery should be accomplished as soon as possible for a given hospital for certain conditions, such as prolapsed cord or uterine rupture. Likewise, it is not always necessary or even desirable to accomplish a cesarean delivery within 30 minutes for some conditions, such as failed induction of labor or failure to progress in labor.

The relationship between timing of acute catastrophic asphyxia and neonatal neurologic outcome is not simple and depends on a number of independent and elusive factors. As seen in the multiple studies summarized previously, adverse neonatal outcome may occur even when the decision-to-delivery interval is only a few minutes.

Conclusions

- The margin between the level of hypoxia that results in cerebral palsy and one that results in perinatal death is narrow. Most cases in which a fetus is subjected to hypoxia of sufficient magnitude to overwhelm the compensatory mechanisms protecting the nervous system result in perinatal death. Of those who survive, only a few develop cerebral palsy.

- As a corollary, most neonates who survive an acute catastrophic hypoxic event would be expected to have normal neurologic outcome.

- Any of the causes of acute catastrophic intrapartum asphyxia may result in neurologic morbidity and sequelae. The result of each insult, however, is not certain and depends on a multitude of poorly understood factors. Clinically, a dose–response association between the magnitude of hypoxia and neurologic damage is not always present. Normal outcomes have been reported following prolonged hypoxia and vice versa.

References

1. Badawi N, Kurinczuk JJ, Keogh JM, Alessandri LM, O'Sullivan F, Burton PR, et al. Antepartum risk factors for newborn encephalopathy: the Western Australian case-control study. BMJ 1998;317: 1549–53. (Level II-2)

2. Nelson KB, Ellenberg JH. Obstetric complications as risk factors for cerebral palsy or seizure disorders. JAMA 1984;251:1843–8. (Level II-2)

3. Nelson KB, Ellenberg JH. Antecedents of cerebral palsy. I. Univariate analysis of risks. Am J Dis Child 1985;139:1031–8. (Level II-2)

4. Nelson KB, Ellenberg JH. Antecedents of cerebral palsy. Multivariate analysis of risk. N Engl J Med 1986;315:81–6. (Level II-2)

5. Torfs CP, van den Berg BJ, Oechsli FW, Cummins S. Prenatal and perinatal factors in the etiology of cerebral palsy. J Pediatr 1990;116:615–9. (Level II-2)

6. Griess FC Jr. Pressure-flow relationship in the gravid uterine vascular bed. Am J Obstet Gynecol 1966; 96:41–7. (Animal study)

7. Martin CB Jr, de Haan J, van der Wildt B, Jongsma HW, Dieleman A, Arts TH. Mechanisms of late deceleration in the fetal heart rate. A study with autonomic blocking agents in fetal lambs. Eur J Obstet Gynecol Reprod Biol 1979;9:361–73. (Animal study)

8. Clark SL, Gimovsky ML, Miller FC. Fetal heart rate response to scalp blood sampling. Am J Obstet Gynecol 1982;144:706–8. (Level II-3)

9. Clark SL, Gimovsky ML, Miller FC. The scalp stimulation test: a clinical alternative to fetal scalp blood sampling. Am J Obstet Gynecol 1984;148:274–7. (Level III)

10. Lee ST, Hon EH. Fetal hemodynamic response to umbilical cord compression. Obstet Gynecol 1963; 22:553–62.(Level III)

11. Kidd LC, Patel N, Smith R. Non-stress antenatal cardiotocography—a prospective randomized clinical trial. Br J Obstet Gynaecol 1985;92:1156–9. (Level II-1)

12. Lumley J, Lester A, Anderson I, Renou P, Wood C. A randomized trial of weekly cardiotocography in high-risk obstetrical patients. Br J Obstet Gynaecol 1983; 90:1018–26. (Level I)

13. Flynn AM, Kelly J, Mansfield H, Needham P, O'Conor M, Viegas O. A randomized controlled trial of non-stress antepartum cardiotocography. Br J Obstet Gynaecol 1982;89:427–33. (Level II-1)

14. Brown VA, Sawers RS, Parsons RJ, Duncan SL, Cooke ID. The value of antenatal cardiotocography in the management of high-risk pregnancy: a randomized controlled trial. Br J Obstet Gynaecol 1982;89: 716–22. (Level I)

15. Neldam S. Fetal movements as an indicator of fetal well being. Lancet 1980;1(8180):1222–4. (Level II-1)

16. Beischer NA, Drew JH, Ashton PW, Oats JN, Gaudry E, Cchen FT, et al. Quality of survival of infants with critical fetal reserve detected by antenatal cardiotocography. Am J Obstet Gynecol 1983;146: 662–70. (Level III)

17. Manning FA, Bondaji N, Harman CR, Casiro O, Menticoglou S, Morrison I, et al. Fetal assessment based on fetal biophysical profile scoring. VIII. The incidence of cerebral palsy in tested and untested perinates. Am J Obstet Gynecol 1998;178:696–706. (Level II-3)

18. Benson RC, Shubeck F, Deutschberger J, Weiss W, Berendes H. Fetal heart rate as a predictor of fetal distress. A report from the collaborative project. Obstet Gynecol 1968;32:259–66. (Level III)

19. Amato JC. Fetal monitoring in a community hospital. A statistical analysis. Obstet Gynecol 1977;50: 269–74. (Level II-2)

20. Chan WH, Paul RH, Toews J. Intrapartum fetal monitoring. Maternal and fetal morbidity and perinatal mortality. Obstet Gynecol 1973;41:7–13. (Level III)

21. Edington PT, Sibanda J, Beard RW. Influence on clinical practice of routine intra-partum fetal monitoring. Br Med J 1975;3:341–3. (Level II-2)

22. Koh KS, Greves D, Yung S, Peddle LJ. Experience with fetal monitoring in a university teaching hospital. Can Med Assoc J 1975;112:455–6, 459–60. (Level III)

23. Lee WK, Baggish MS. The effect of unselected intrapartum fetal monitoring. Obstet Gynecol 1976;47: 516–20. (Level II-2)

24. Paul RH, Huey JR, Yaeger CF. Clinical fetal monitoring: its effect on cesarean section rate and perinatal mortality: five-year trends. Postgrad Med 1977;61: 160–6. (Level II-2)

25. Shenker L, Post RC, Seiler JS. Routine electronic monitoring of the fetal heart rate and uterine activity during labor. Obstet Gynecol 1975;46:185–9. (Level III)

26. Tutera G, Newman RL. Fetal monitoring: its effect on perinatal mortality and cesarean section rates and its complications. Am J Obstet Gynecol 1975;122: 750–4. (Level II-2)

27. Quilligan EJ, Paul RH. Fetal monitoring: is it worth it? Obstet Gynecol 1975;45:96–100. (Level III)

28. Haverkamp AD, Thompson HE, McFee JG, Cetrulo C. The evaluation of continuous fetal heart rate monitoring in high-risk pregnancy. Am J Obstet Gynecol 1976;125:310–20. (Level II-1)

29. Haverkamp AD, Orleans M, Langendoerfer S, McFee J, Murphy J, Thompson HE. A controlled trial of differential effects of intrapartum fetal monitoring. Am J Obstet Gynecol 1979;134:399–412. (Level II-1)

30. Kelso IM, Parsons RJ, Lawrence GF, Arora SS, Edmonds DK, Cooke ID. An assessment of continuous fetal heart rate monitoring in labor. A randomized trial. Am J Obstet Gynecol 1978;131:526–32. (Level II-1)

31. Mc Donald D, Grant A, Sheridan-Periera M, Boylan P, Chalmers I. The Dublin randomized controlled trial of intrapartum fetal heart rate monitoring. Am J Obstet Gynecol 1985;152:524–39. (Level I)

32. Renou P, Chang A, Anderson I, Wood C. Controlled trial of fetal intensive care. Am J Obstet Gynecol 1976;126:470–6. (Level I)

33. Wood C, Renou P, Oates J, Farrell E, Beischer N, Anderson I. A controlled trial of fetal heart rate monitoring in a low-risk population. Am J Obstet Gynecol 1981;141:527–34. (Level I)

34. Banta HD, Thacker SB. Costs and benefits of electronic fetal monitoring: a review of the literature. Hyattsville (MD): National Center for Health Services Research, U.S. Department of Health, Education, and Welfare; 1979 April. DHEW publication no (PHS) 79-3245. (Level III)

35. Hobbins JC, Freeman R, Queenan JT. The fetal monitoring debate. Pediatrics 1979;63:942–51. (Level III)

36. Grant A, O'Brien N, Joy MT, Hennessy E, MacDonald D. Cerebral palsy among children born during the Dublin randomized trial of intrapartum monitoring. Lancet 1989;2:1233–6. (Level I)

37. Grant A. Epidemiological principles for the evaluation of monitoring programs—the Dublin experience. Clin Invest Med 1993;16:119–58. (Level III)

38. Thacker SB, Stroup DF, Peterson HB. Efficacy and safety of intrapartum electronic fetal monitoring: an update. Obstet Gynecol 1995;86:613–20. (Level III)

39. Stalnaker BL, Maher JE, Kleinman GE, Macksey JM, Fishman LA, Rernard JM. Characteristics of successful claims for payment by the Florida Neurologic Injury Compensation Association Fund. Am J Obstet Gynecol 1997;177:268–71; discussion 271–3. (Level III)

40. Schifrin BS, Dame L. Fetal heart rate patterns. Prediction of Apgar score. JAMA 1972;219:1322–5. (Level II-2)

41. Nelson KB, Dambrosia JM, Ting TY, Grether JK. Uncertain value of electronic fetal monitoring in predicting cerebral palsy. N Engl J Med 1996;334:613–8. (Level II-2)

42. Goodwin TM, Milner-Masterson L, Paul RH. Elimination of fetal scalp blood sampling on a large clinical service. Obstet Gynecol 1994;83:971–4. (Level II-2)

43. Garite TJ, Dildy GA, McNamara H, Nageotte MP, Boehm FH, Dellinger EH, et al. A multicenter controlled trial of fetal pulse oximetry in the intrapartum management of nonreassuring fetal heart rate patterns. Am J Obstet Gynecol 2000;183:1049–58. (Level I)

44. Freeman R. Intrapartum fetal monitoring—a disappointing story [editorial]. N Eng J Med 1990;322:624–6. (Level III)

45. Hagberg B, Hagberg G, Olow I. The changing panorama of cerebral palsy in Sweden. IV. Epidemiologic trends 1959–78. Acta Paediatr Scand 1984;73:433–40. (Level II-3)

46. Stanley FJ, Watson L. The cerebral palsies in western Australia: trends, 1968 to 1981. Am J Obstet Gynecol 1988;158:89–93. (Level II-3)

47. Zuspan FP, Quilligan EJ, Iams JD, van Geijn HP. Predictors of intrapartum fetal distress: the role of electronic fetal monitoring. Report of the National Institute of Child Health and Human Development Consensus Development Task Force. Am J Obstet Gynecol 1979;135:287–91. (Level III)

48. Roland EH, Poskitt K, Rodriguez E, Lupton BA, Hill A. Perinatal hypoxic-ischemic thalamic injury: clinical features and neuroimaging. Ann Neurol 1998;44:161–6. (Level III)

49. Pasternak JF, Gorey MT. The syndrome of acute near-total intrauterine asphyxia in the term infant. Pediatr Neurol 1998;18:391–8. (Level III)

50. Myers RE. Fetal asphyxia due to umbilical cord compression. Metabolic and brain pathologic consequences. Biol Neonate 1975;26:21–43. (Animal study)

51. Phelan JP, Ahn MO, Korst L, Martin GI, Wang YM. Intrapartum fetal asphyxial brain injury with absent multiorgan system dysfunction. J Matern Fetal Med 1998;7:19–22. (Level III)

52. Keunen H, Blanco CE, van Reempts JL, Hasaart TH. Absence of neuronal damage after umbilical cord occlusion of 10, 15, and 20 minutes in midgestation fetal sheep. Am J Obstet Gynecol 1997;176:515–20. (Animal study)

53. De Haan HH, Gunn AJ, Williams CE, Gluckman PD. Brief repeated umbilical cord occlusions cause sustained cytotoxic cerebral edema and focal infarcts in near-term fetal lambs. Pediatr Res 1997;41:96–104. (Animal study)

54. Myers RE. Threshold values of oxygen deficiency leading to cardiovascular and brain pathological changes in term monkey fetuses. Adv Exp Med Biol 1973;37:1047–53. (Animal study)

55. Myers RE. Two patterns of perinatal brain damage and their conditions of occurrence. Am J Obstet Gynecol 1972;112:246–76. (Animal study)

56. Mirsky AF, Orren MM, Stanton L, Fullerton BC, Harris S, Myers RE. Auditory evoked potentials and auditory behavior following prenatal and perinatal asphyxia in rhesus monkeys. Dev Psychobiol 1979;12:369–79. (Animal study)

57. Myers RE. Brain damage induced by umbilical cord compression at different gestational ages in monkeys. In: Goldsmith EI, Moor-Jankowski J, editors. Medical Primatology Conference on experimental medicine and surgery in primates. New York: Karger, Basel; 1970. p. 394–425. (Animal study)

58. Wagner KR, Ting P, Westfall MV, Yamaguchi S, Bacher JD, Myers RE. Brain metabolic correlates of hypoxic-ischemic cerebral necrosis in mid-gestational sheep fetuses: significance of hypotension. J Cereb Blood Flow Metab 1986;6:425–34. (Animal study)

59. Roohey T, Raju TN, Moustogiannis AN. Animal models for the study of perinatal hypoxic-ischemic encephalopathy: a critical analysis. Early Hum Dev 1997;47:115–46. (Animal study)

60. Ranck JB Jr, Windle WF. Brain damage in the monkey, Macaca mulatta, by asphyxia neonatorum. Exp Neurol 1959;1:130–54. (Animal study)

61. Nicolaides KH, Economides DL, Soothill PW. Blood gases, pH and lactate in appropriate- and small-for-gestational-age fetuses. Am J Obstet Gynecol 1989;161:996–1001. (Level II-2)

62. Soothill PW, Nicolaides KH, Rodeck CH, Campbell S. Effect of gestational age on fetal and intervillous blood gas and acid-base values in human pregnancy. Fetal Ther 1986;1:168–75. (Level II-3)

63. Soothill PW, Nicolaides KH, Rodeck CH, Gamsu H. Blood gases and acid-base status of the human second-trimester fetus. Obstet Gynecol 1986;68:173–6. (Level II-3)

64. Weiner CP. The relationship between the umbilical artery systolic/diastolic ratio and umbilical blood gas measurements in specimens obtained by cordocentesis. Am J Obstet Gynecol 1990;162:1198–1202. (Level II-3)

65. Weiner CP, Sipes SL, Wenstrom K. The effect of fetal age upon normal fetal laboratory values and venous pressure. Obstet Gynecol 1992;79:713–8. (Level II-3)

66. Vintzileos AM, Egan JF, Campbell WA, Rodis JF, Scorza WE, Fleming AD, et al. Asphyxia at birth as determined by cord blood pH measurements in preterm and term gestations: correlation with neonatal outcome. J Matern Fetal Med 1992;1:7–13. (Level II-2)

67. Richardson B, Nodwell A, Webster K, Alshimmiri M, Gagnon R, Natale R. Fetal oxygen saturation and fractional extraction at birth and the relationship to measures of acidosis. Am J Obstet Gynecol 1998;178:572–9. (Level II-2)

68. Woo JS, Ngan YS, Ma HK. Prolapse and presentation of the umbilical cord. Aust N Z J Obstet Gynaecol 1983;23:142–5. (Level II-2)

69. Niswander KR, Friedman EA, Hoover DB, Pietrowski H, Westphal M. Fetal morbidity following potentially anoxigenic obstetric conditions. III. Prolapse of the umbilical cord. Am J Obstet Gynecol 1966;95:853–9. (Level II-2)

70. Niswander KR, Friedman EA, Hoover DB, Pietrowski H, Westphal M. Fetal morbidity following potentially anoxigenic obstetric conditions. IV. Occult prolapse of the umbilical cord. Am J Obstet Gynecol 1966;95:1099–103. (Level II-2)

71. Murphy DJ, MacKenzie IZ. The mortality and morbidity associated with umbilical cord prolapse. Br J Obstet Gynaecol 1995;102:826–30. (Level II-2)

72. Hope P, Breslin S, Lamont L, Lucas A, Martin D, Moore I, et al. Fatal shoulder dystocia: a review of 56 cases reported to the Confidential Enquiry into Stillbirths and Deaths in Infancy. Br J Obstet Gynaecol 1998;105:1256–61. (Level III)

73. Leung AS, Leung EK, Paul RH. Uterine rupture after previous cesarean delivery: maternal and fetal consequences. Am J Obstet Gynecol 1993;169:945–50. (Level III)

74. Menihan CA. Uterine rupture in women attempting a vaginal birth following prior cesarean birth. J Perinatol 1998;18:440–3. (Level III)

75. Clark SL, Hankins GD, Dudley DA, Dildy GA, Porter TF. Amniotic fluid embolism: analysis of the national registry. Am J Obstet Gynecol 1995;172:1158–67; discussion 1167–9. (Level II-2)

76. Katz VL, Dotters DJ, Droegemueller W. Perimortem cesarean delivery. Obstet Gynecol 1986;68:571–6. (Level III)

77. Lopez-Zeno JA, Carlo WA, O'Grady JP, Fanaroff AA. Infant survival following delayed postmortem cesarean delivery. Obstet Gynecol 1990;76:991–2. (Level III)

78. American Academy of Pediatrics, American College of Obstetricians and Gynecologists. Intrapartum and postpartum care of women. In: Guidelines for perinatal care. 5th ed. Elk Grove Village (IL): AAP; Washington (DC): ACOG; 2002. p. 125–61. (Level III)

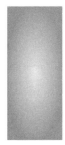

CHAPTER 4

FETAL CONSIDERATIONS

Neurologic Outcome in Multiple Pregnancy

Multiple Pregnancy and Cerebral Palsy

An association between multiple gestation and cerebral palsy in resulting off-spring has been established for some time. In 1897, Sigmund Freud reported twin birth to be higher than birth asphyxia or preterm delivery in a list of causes of spastic diplegia (1). Since then, many studies on the etiology of cerebral palsy have noted a greater than expected contribution from children of multiple gestations (2–11). In these reports, the prevalence of cerebral palsy in multiple pregnancy ranges from 5.4% (3) to 10.8% (2). The study design in many of these reports is not of the highest scientific quality; however, the fact that the principal finding is so similar in all of them lends support to the veracity of this association.

Studies of series of multiple pregnancies with cerebral palsy have since been performed (12, 13), and epidemiologic studies have investigated the prevalence of cerebral palsy in multiple gestations (14–20). Despite potential regional differences, differences in standards of medical care, and possible population ascertainment bias, the most reported prevalences of cerebral palsy in multiple pregnancies are remarkably consistent (ranging from 6.7 to 12.6 per 1,000 surviving infants). The most frequently quoted incidence of cerebral palsy for twins is approximately 7 per 1,000. Some of the variation in reported statistics depends on the population studied and the method of identification used. In one study, when the prevalence was calculated per pregnancy (rather than per live birth), the prevalence of cerebral palsy was as high as 13.2 per 1,000 in twins and 75.9 per 1,000 in triplets (17). Another group of investigators reported the risk of producing at least one child with cerebral palsy from one pregnancy to be 15 per 1,000 for twins, 80 per 1,000 for triplets, and 429 per 1,000 for quadruplets (20). Of these quoted, only one included a control group of twins (10). The comparison showed that low birth weight, first born birth order, and uniovularity were significantly higher in twins with cerebral palsy than in twins without cerebral palsy (controls).

Preterm Delivery

Because cerebral palsy is associated with preterm delivery, and because multiple pregnancy is strongly associated with preterm delivery, it is intuitive that an association of cerebral palsy with multiple pregnancy should exist. Indeed the prevalence of cerebral palsy is greater in multiple gestations that result in babies of lower birth weights (15, 17). Furthermore, in very-low-birth weight babies, there is no difference in rates of cerebral palsy between singletons and twins (14–18, 21). Clearly, at very low birth weights, the effect is caused more by the extreme prematurity than the plurality of the gestation. Although multiple pregnancy has been reported to be an independent risk factor for cerebral palsy at all gestational ages (19), more investigators have found this to be true at higher birth weights (14–18, 21). The risk of cerebral palsy has been reported as 3–3.8 times more likely in twins with birth weights more than 2,500 g when compared with singletons matched for birth weight (14, 17). In another study, the relative risk (RR) for cerebral palsy was 4.5 (95% confidence interval [CI], 1.4–14.4) in a similar comparison; when twins were compared with singletons of more than 37 weeks of gestation, the RR of cerebral palsy was 6.3 (95% CI, 2–20) (19). Therefore, there is a significant risk of cerebral palsy in offspring of multiple gestations that is not simply related to the greater incidence of preterm delivery in such pregnancies.

Zygosity and Chorionicity

Some studies have associated monozygosity with neurologic impairment in twin gestations when compared with dizygosity (13). Also, monochorionicity is much more strongly associated with neurologic impairment than dichorionicity (odds ratio [OR], 6; 95% CI, 1.7–21.3 for cerebral palsy or severe mental retardation for monochorionic compared with dichorionic gestations) (22, 23).

Birth Order

Although much of the literature suggests no correlation between birth order and long-term neurologic impairment (5–7, 11, 13, 24), one paper (10) reported that twins with cerebral palsy are predominantly first born and the nonsurvivors are predominantly second born.

Sex

Some investigators have noted a preponderance of male infants from multiple gestations affected with cerebral palsy from multiple gestations (10, 14). However, other studies have reported the sex-associated risk of cerebral palsy to be equal (9, 13, 17). To date, no conclusive evidence of a sex-associated risk can be drawn from the literature.

Concordance

Although a considerable amount of medical literature is devoted to the importance of weight discordance in multiple gestations, there is remarkably little published on its effect on long-term neurologic function (12, 17, 24). One early study noted unaffected twins were heavier than twins affected with cerebral palsy by an average of 2.8 oz (12). If the analysis was limited to those twins with quadriplegia, the unaffected twins were an average of 8 oz heavier. Another publication noted that in cases of discordant birth weights, the affected twin was heavier in 20 (66%) cases, lighter in nine (30%), and the same in one (3%) (17). In a Swedish series of 5,382 twins, the larger twin in the pair had a significantly higher incidence of cerebral palsy than the smaller one (RR, 2.6, 95% CI, 1.4–4.8) (24). Therefore, although in obstetric practice it is traditionally thought that the smaller twin is at greater risk, the limited amount of published evidence suggests this is not true for cerebral palsy.

Intrauterine Demise of One Twin

In one of the first series of children with cerebral palsy, it was noted that among 19 sets of twins affected with cerebral palsy, in 10 cases the co-twin was either a stillbirth or died shortly after birth (3). A substantial incidence of stillbirth in the co-twin of children affected with cerebral palsy was reported in other research (10, 25) and reproduced in some epidemiologic studies (14, 13, 17, 18). In a case series in which one twin had died in utero, the incidence of mental retardation was 40% and that of seizures was 20% (13). Other studies have found the incidence of cerebral palsy in cases in which one twin died in utero from four times (17) to 15 times (18) higher than when both twins survived. One study of a large cohort of twins noted the incidence of cerebral palsy in the surviving twin was 121 per 1,000 (14): 13 times higher than gestations in which both twins survived, and 100 times higher than in singletons. A series of 79 sets of triplets noted seven cases in which one fetus died in utero (17) and found a prevalence of cerebral palsy of 154 per 1,000 among those who survived to 1 year, compared with 29 per 1,000 when all of the triplets were born alive. Because of the small numbers of cases studied, caution should be exercised in interpreting these data.

Two large epidemiologic studies have investigated the specific issue of long-term follow-up after antenatal death of a twin (26, 27). In the earlier of these two studies (1973–1980), long-term follow-up of twin gestations in which one twin had died was compared with twin pregnancies of similar birth weight and date of delivery (26). The study group in which one twin had died had a greater proportion of monozygous twins than the control group (69.5% versus 45.4%). The study group also had a greater incidence of cerebral palsy or mental retardation (4.6%) in the surviving twin. A later study (1993–1995) identified 613 twin pregnancies in the United Kingdom in which one fetus had died in utero (27). Long-term follow-up investigation revealed the overall prevalence of cerebral palsy in the live-born twin was 83 per 1,000 (95% CI, 57–117), an increase of 40-fold over the background population prevalence of cerebral palsy in England.

The latter study compared same-sex and different-sex pairs in an attempt to differentiate between monozygous and dizygous twins. The prevalence of cerebral palsy in same-sex twins was 106 per 1,000 (95% CI, 70–150). For different-sex twins, the prevalence of cerebral palsy was 29 per 1,000 (95% CI, 6–83). Using same-sex and different-sex as a surrogate for zygosity, there is likely to be a much greater incidence of neurologic impairment in a monozygotic pregnancy, which most likely results from the presence of a monochorionic placentation.

Most reported cases of intrauterine demise of one twin are managed expectantly (28–41). In some series, both expectant and emergency delivery strategies have been pursued (42–46). Even in some cases in which emergency cesarean delivery was performed the same day as diagnosis of the demise of one twin, neurologic impairment still ensued in the survivor (42, 43). Although close fetal surveillance seems intuitive, it may be misleading, as normal fetal heart rate patterns and biophysical profile scores have been documented even in the presence of multicystic encephalomalacia (43). Thus, in most preterm cases of death in utero, caused by the uncertainty of both the time of demise and possible neurologic sequelae, expectant management is most appropriate. No strategies have been identified that allow the clinician to alter these outcomes.

Monochorionic Placentation

As noted, monozygotic and monochorionic twin gestations have a worse prognosis than their dizygotyic and dichorionic counterparts in terms of long-term neurologic impairment. Furthermore, the risk of neurologic injury is highest in monochorionic twins when one twin dies, and this risk is much higher than the risk of injury in monochorionic twins without demise (29, 31, 35, 38–40, 43, 46, 47). Although the increased incidence of neurologic impairment seen in monozygotic and monochorionic twin gestations in which both twins survive may be caused by vascular anastomoses, it also may be caused by many other factors, such as intrauterine growth restriction (IUGR), complications of a velamentous cord insertion, preterm rupture of membranes, delivery, or any injuries that may lead to neurologic impairment of the fetus or infant (22, 48–51).

An investigation into the antenatal origin of neurologic damage in multiple gestations used ultrasound assessments of the neonatal brain within 3 days of birth (25). Cerebral atrophy and white-matter cavitation were used as indicators of white-matter necrosis. A total of 101 infants (89 twins and 12 triplets) were studied. Fourteen babies (13.8%) were diagnosed as having antenatal necrosis of cerebral white matter. The incidence of white-matter necrosis was greater in monochorionic as opposed to dichorionic infants (30% versus 3.3%; $P < 0.001$). In this study, cerebral white-matter necrosis was associated with polyhydramnios, intrauterine death of a co-twin, hydrops, and placental vascular connections (particularly vein-to-vein anastomosis).

Many pathologic lesions can be found in the surviving twin following an intrauterine demise in a monochorionic pregnancy, but renal cortical necrosis and multicystic encephalomalacia are particularly remarkable (36, 39–43, 46). Possible contributing factors include IUGR, marginal and velamentous umbilical cord insertions, extreme fetal growth discordance, and preterm delivery. However, the typical findings of renal cortical necrosis and multicystic encephalomalacia in monochorionic twin gestations point to a common pathologic process. Both circumstantial and objective evidence exist to suggest this mechanism results from the presence of vascular connections in monochorionic placentation.

It has been known for many years that the death of one twin in utero may have effects on the other in the setting of monochorionic placentation. In 1882, Fredereich Schatz documented the existence of vascular connections within monochorionic placentas (52). Abnormal findings in surviving twins of an intrauterine demise in monochorionic twin gestations may be related to this vascular architecture. However, the mechanism could result from transfusion of products through the placental vascular connections or from abnormal hemodynamics secondary to the existence of the connections themselves.

In an attempt to understand the mechanism, funipuncture was carried out on surviving twins who were being expectantly managed after the intrauterine demise of their co-twin (53). In 5 of 7 cases, the placenta was monochorionic, and 3 of these 5 had cerebral anomalies postnatally. The fetal blood samples did not reveal coagulopathy in any of the surviving twins but did reveal anemia in three cases (two monochorionic, the other of unknown chorionicity). These findings suggest that the possible mechanism for the abnormalities found in the surviving twin (after the death of a co-twin in cases of monochorionic placentation) is the hemorrhage of the survivor into the dead co-twin. This would lead to a hypotensive episode and consequently, tissue hypoxia and infarction in the survivor. This can be thought of as a "capacitance" effect of the dead twin on its living counterpart.

An extreme case of placental vascular communication is in twin-to-twin transfusion syndrome. Twin-to-twin transfusion syndrome is a complication of monochorionic twin gestation in which blood is shunted from one twin to the other through uncompensated placental vascular anastomoses. Three strategies to improve outcome in twin-to twin transfusion are 1) serial amnioreduction, 2) laser ablation of communicating vessels, and 3) septostomy of communicating vessels (54–65). Although some studies report that serial amnioreduction may improve survivability, the benefit of the other two strategies has not been determined. Only one publication has reported on long-term outcome in twin-to-twin transfusion syndrome (60). This study, which followed a cohort of twin gestations (beyond age 2 years) with the syndrome who were treated with aggressive amniocentesis, showed that two of 42 infants (4.7%) developed cerebral palsy.

Conclusions

- Multiple gestation is an independent risk factor for cerebral palsy and long-term neurologic impairment.

- The risk for cerebral palsy and long-term neurologic impairment is significantly higher for monochorionic twins.

- In cases of intrauterine fetal demise in twins, there is an increased risk of neurologic compromise in the surviving fetus. This risk is substantially increased in cases of monochorionic presentation.

- Currently, there are no identified strategies that allow the clinician to affect the outcomes.

Intrauterine Growth Restriction and Neonatal Encephalopathy

Definition and Characterization

The term "intrauterine growth restriction" often is used synonymously with small-for-gestational age (SGA). However the term IUGR connotes an intrauterine pathophysiologic process resulting in restriction of fetal growth, while SGA refers more simply to a statistical grouping of newborns. Practically speaking, there is considerable overlap of the two terms; however, at a conceptual level, the distinction between the two may be important. If there is to be any reduction in the morbidity and mortality of IUGR as well as a better understanding of links to long-term outcome, this poorly defined entity must be more fully understood.

The primary classifications of the newborn rely on a statistical approach, relating birth weight to gestational age. Only newborns with a birth weight greater than two standard deviations below the mean for any gestational age (less than 2.5th percentile) are truly SGA. However, because many share common similar problems, all newborns with birth weights below the 10th percentile for gestational age are regarded as SGA (66). Modern national standard weights for each week of gestation are available for singleton male and female newborns (67).

There is debate about the relevant clinical percentile threshold associated with increased risk for neonatal encephalopathy. Adverse perinatal outcome is generally confined to those newborns with birth weights below the fifth percentile and in most cases below the third percentile (68, 69). A large, population-based, case–control study supports a significant increase in RR for newborn encephalopathy in infants with birth weights less than the third percentile when compared with birth weights between the third and ninth percentiles (adjusted OR, 38.23 and 4.37 respectively) and when compared to birth weights above the ninth percentile (adjusted OR, 1.54) (68).

Statistically, 10% of newborns should fall below the 10th percentile, regardless of medical condition or intervention. Some reflect growth restriction, while others may simply reflect biologic diversity. Most standardized "growth curves" are in fact static, cross-sectional measurements collected near the time of birth and do not represent serial or precise measurements in the same subject over time.

Descriptive Classifications

Etiology, the time of onset, and the duration of growth restriction determine the pattern and severity of diminished growth. Therefore, other classification schemes have been developed to characterize the heterogeneous group of newborns included under the term SGA, as well as some appropriate-growth-for-gestational-age newborns that have had restricted growth. Each system offers insight into the determination of the origin, the counseling to be offered, as well as the long-term outcome of the individual newborn.

Total reliance on gestational age and birth weight ignores differences in body length and size as well as relative head size. Not all SGA newborns are growth restricted. Some SGA newborns represent the normal distribution of neonatal weight among a normal base population (70). In contrast, a fetus whose growth stops or slows but is delivered before its weight crosses below the 10th percentile, should be considered to be subjected to a growth-restricting process, even if its weight is appropriate for gestational age. Practically speaking, it is reasonable to regard such a newborn as "at risk" even if above an arbitrary percentile. The dilemma, of course, is that there is no reliable way to determine that a fetus born at the 25th percentile was genetically destined to be born at the 80th percentile.

Many newborns, particularly those born at term or beyond, demonstrate evidence of weight loss and should be considered within the spectrum of IUGR, even if their birth weight is greater than 2,500 g (66). There is currently no satisfactory means, except perhaps by the ponderal index, to assign an IUGR diagnosis if the newborn weighs more than 2,500 g (71).

Historically, fetal growth restriction has been further divided by some into symmetric and asymmetric types. This is to distinguish between early- and late-onset impairment of growth (72).

Asymmetric Intrauterine Growth Restriction

Newborns in this descriptive category fall into two subcategories. One is characterized by weight at or below the 10th percentile, but with head circumference and length above the 10th percentile. These newborns have the potential for normal growth and development, but are potentially more likely to demonstrate intrapartum fetal heart rate alterations and to be more vulnerable to perinatal hypoxia/metabolic acidemia. Also vulnerable and frequently overlooked are similar newborns at term or beyond that demonstrate evidence of recent weight loss (wasting), such as loss of subcutaneous tissue and associated loose skin folds (66, 71).

Symmetric Intrauterine Growth Restriction

In this group, both the length and birth weight are below the 10th percentile. Although this subcategory is commonly associated with so-called "intrinsic" fetal problems and early onset of growth restriction, these associations do not always hold true. If substrate deprivation is prolonged, it may ultimately affect length and head circumference as well as present a picture of symmetric IUGR.

Ponderal Index

One method to characterize the newborn growth pattern is the ponderal index (73, 74). Care must be taken to measure newborn length, because it is cubed in the ponderal index formula:

$$\frac{\text{Birthweight}^2 \text{ (g)}}{\text{Crown-heel length (cm)}^3 \times 100}$$

Clinically, the ponderal index is useful as a means to further subclassify IUGR as symmetric or asymmetric and to identify wasted newborns (66). In addition, SGA neonates with a low ponderal index have a significantly increased risk of complications when compared with SGA neonates with a normal ponderal index (75).

Neonatal Encephalopathy and Cerebral Palsy

Most IUGR or SGA newborns, even if markedly SGA, do not sustain developmental handicaps or cerebral palsy. In fact, most newborns destined to develop cerebral palsy are of normal birth weight.

Cerebral palsy is more common in preterm infants than IUGR infants. Although IUGR is closely linked to cerebral palsy, the role of IUGR as an independent predictor is not completely defined (76). In large part the uncertainty arises from the inherent power limitations imposed by addressing an infrequent outcome (cerebral palsy) in a 10% heterogeneous subset of newborns (if SGA is used as the criteria for IUGR). By definition, 10% of newborns will have birth weights below the 10th percentile. As an example, IUGR can occur in newborns with a birth weight at the 15th to 20th percentile whose genetic predisposition would have intended birth at the 90th percentile in a neutral environment. Furthermore, while a 10th percentile cutoff may be only marginally relevant, it is a strategic device to ensure inclusion of at-risk newborns.

Further complicating the issue is the complex nature of the association of IUGR with cerebral palsy. Most reported studies employ a retrospective, case–control approach. Many factors associated with or considered to serve as direct causes of IUGR also may have an independent direct effect on neurologic development. Conditions in which IUGR/SGA does not lie within the causation pathway but in which cerebral palsy, neurodevelopmental handicap, and IUGR may instead be the result of common antecedents are as follows:

- Cytogenetic abnormalities—many are SGA and have neurodevelopmental handicaps. In such cases SGA is not the cause, but, like the handicap, a product.

- Congenital infections

- Structural abnormalities

- Substance abuse (alcohol and drugs)

- Coagulation disorders

The linkage between cerebral palsy and IUGR is incompletely established, even when hypoxia/metabolic acidosis is considered. Two questions remain: Is the IUGR newborn who does not experience hypoxia at increased risk for developmental handicap/cerebral palsy? Are the handicaps arising in IUGR newborns who experience hypoxia the product of the hypoxia or the result of IUGR? If IUGR is the result of diminished provision of nutrients and oxygen by the placenta, diminished oxygenation during labor is more likely than in the normally grown fetus. Clinically significant fetal hypoxemia and related acidemia are more common in SGA newborns (77). Unfortunately, studies addressing this issue are limited by lack of consensus, universal definitions, or criteria for what constitutes fetal hypoxia, asphyxia, and acidemia. As a result, the precise nature of the link between IUGR and cerebral palsy as well as other neurologic sequelae is debatable (70).

Some insight into the role of hypoxemia is provided in a study of data from the National Collaborative Perinatal Project, which found infants with IUGR (symmetric and asymmetric) who did not have hypoxemia-related risk factors were not at greater risk for neurologic morbidity or cerebral palsy than infants without IUGR. However, newborns with IUGR and hypoxia-related factors were more likely to have later neurologic deficits than were their counterparts without IUGR (49). Other investigators have similarly concluded clinically significant hypoxia-acidosis causes at least part of the increase in cerebral palsy seen in term IUGR/SGA newborns (78). Low-ponderal-index SGA infants also generally have normal outcomes unless labor is complicated by clinically significant metabolic acidosis.

Two reports suggest a mechanism that accounts for the increased risk of cerebral palsy associated with IUGR (79, 80). An increased frequency of IUGR and oligohydramnios is associated with white-matter damage, which suggests chronic fetal hypoxia that results in oligohydramnios also may result in fetal cerebral ischemia, which in turn results in the white-matter lesion.

Many studies of newborn encephalopathy were limited to newborns that showed so-called signs of hypoxia and ischemia during labor. Increased insight is provided by a population-based, unmatched control investigation of the relative role of a wider range of potential causes of moderate and severe encephalopathy in term newborns, arising from before conception until after birth (68). After adjusting for the presence of multiple known risk factors, newborn encephalopathy was most strongly associated with IUGR at less than or equal to the third percentile. The authors emphasized the importance of their selection of a study population by gestational age rather than birth weight, because birth weight would have underestimated the impact of IUGR.

Each cause of growth restriction may differ in its relative impact on the causation of encephalopathy or in predisposing a fetus to the damaging impact of an intermediate factor. Preeclampsia is a common cause of IUGR and has a strong independent RR for encephalopathy (68, 81).

Fetal growth restriction (defined as birth weight less than the 10th percentile for gestation, as a biologic variable) has been shown to have an adverse impact on behavioral characteristics of attention and learning, causing inattention and learning deficits. A study of high-risk newborns with growth restriction that excluded children with genetic or major organ system malformations found 48% (37/77) had learning deficits at ages 9–11 years (82). There also is a significant independent relationship with environmental factors, such as parental education, father's occupation, social setting, and heredity (82).

A strong association exists for IUGR/SGA newborns born after 33 weeks of gestation with spastic cerebral palsy. The association is most marked in newborns who are short, thin, and have a small head size (83). Newborns above or below the 10th percentile for weight but with an abnormal ponderal index also are at risk for spastic cerebral palsy (84). Interestingly, IUGR also is a significant risk factor for later chronic hypertension, ischemic heart disease, diabetes, and obstructive lung disease, suggesting that a phenomenon of "programming" during a critical period of fetal growth and development in an adverse fetal environment may be operative in the promotion of multiple long-term consequences (85).

The impact of IUGR/SGA status in the preterm newborn is difficult to decipher. In general, when study cohorts are defined by birthweight, preterm SGA newborns have less cerebral palsy than preterm appropriate growth for gestational age newborns. In contrast, when cohorts are defined by gestational age, SGA newborns have similar or higher associated rates of cerebral palsy (70). Other investigators have failed to confirm this finding (86). Preeclampsia, a common association with preterm SGA/IUGR, may play a protective role (87). The nature and mechanism of potential protection is complicated by associated confounders, including the use of magnesium sulfate, which may independently provide a protective effect (88), although this latter hypothesis has rarely been called into question (89, 90). In one study, SGA (<10th percentile) newborns with birth weights less than 1,500 g were not at greater risk for cerebral palsy than matched controls with appropriate growth for gestational age or birthweight (87, 88).

It is likely the adverse developmental outcomes associated with IUGR/SGA in otherwise healthy newborns are the result of nonnutritional causes. Data from studies of the siege of Leningrad (91) and the Dutch famine (92) collected during World War II suggest maternal intake must be reduced to below 1,500 kcal per day before measurable impact on birth weight becomes evident. These data provide significant evidence that nutritional deficiency associated with IUGR is unlikely to play a causal role when acting alone. It is not clear, however, how much of the effect on birth weight was the result of IUGR and how much the result of preterm delivery.

Conclusions

- Data from randomized controlled trials find no interventions other than delivery beneficial in preventing or treating IUGR. Even if maternal medical conditions are thought to be the cause of IUGR, there is no evidence that changes in maternal medical management, other than delivery, alter outcome.

- The etiology and manifestations of IUGR are numerous, and the causation of IUGR is relevant in any attempt to establish the causation of the outcome observed, eg, neonatal encephalopathy.

Meconium and Cerebral Palsy

Like the Apgar score, meconium staining of the amniotic fluid has been used as a marker for newborn asphyxia or hypoxia. However, also like the Apgar score, it has proved to be a poor predictor of long-term neurologic disability, especially cerebral palsy, in the term infant. One study of more than 42,000 term singleton newborns did find a significantly higher incidence of low 1- and 5-minute Apgar scores, umbilical artery blood pH of 7 or less, and seizures on the first day of life among subjects where meconium was detected in the amniotic fluid (93). However, there was no long-term follow-up of these newborns. Another study reported meconium-stained amniotic fluid may be associated with elevated erythropoietin levels in the fetus, possibly suggesting chronic hypoxia (94). Other research found no significant correlation between meconium in the amniotic fluid and fetal acid–base status (95). Although there might be a slight increase in cerebral palsy associated with meconium-stained amniotic fluid, 99.6% of newborns who weighed more than 2,500 g at birth and had meconium staining did not have cerebral palsy (96, 97). A review comparing 46 children (≥2,500 g at birth) with spastic cerebral palsy with 378 controls found no association between meconium-stained amniotic fluid and cerebral palsy (98). Although meconium-induced vasoconstriction of the umbilical cord vessels has been postulated as a cause of fetal hypoxia, this has not been confirmed by scientific studies on intact umbilical cord segments (99–102).

Meconium staining of the amniotic fluid is primarily gestational-age dependent and is uncommon in the preterm infant. It is important to note discolored fluid is not necessarily meconium and may be old blood (103) or the result of infection with Listeria (104, 105). Meconium-stained amniotic fluid may be a risk factor for bacterial invasion of the amniotic cavity (106).

Conclusions

- Passage of meconium usually is a physiologic function and is rarely a marker of an adverse event.
- The incidence of meconium-stained amniotic fluid increases with gestational age.
- Meconium stained amniotic fluid is a poor predictor of long-term neurologic outcome.

The Relative Impact of Postterm Birth Versus Postmaturity on Subsequent Neonatal Encephalopathy and Cerebral Palsy

An Agency for Healthcare Research and Quality technology assessment confirms historical estimates that perinatal mortality rates increase substantially after 41 weeks of gestation (107). An early retrospective study addressing the outcome of postterm newborns weighing less than 2,500 g reported their mortality rate to be seven times that of all postterm newborns (108).

Prolonged pregnancy continues to pose a risk for nonreassuring fetal heart rate patterns and metabolic acidosis, especially in the presence of oligohydramnios. Of pregnancies extending beyond 41 weeks, 23% and 4% of newborns weigh more than 4,000 g and 4,500 g, respectively (109). The association of postterm pregnancy with birth weight greater than 4,500–5,000 g also poses an increased risk for shoulder dystocia and brachial plexus palsy.

Conclusions derived from some early reports of long-term outcomes of pregnancies thought to be prolonged or postterm must be interpreted with caution. Gestational age was commonly overestimated before the widespread use of ultrasonography (110, 111).

A large, population-based, case–control study identified a significant increase in RR for encephalopathy with each week after 39 weeks of gestation. Compared with newborns delivered at 39 weeks of gestation, the adjusted RR increased to 1.41 at 40 weeks, 3.34 at 41 weeks, and 13.2 at 42 weeks of gestation (68).

Most reports addressing the development of infants from prolonged or postterm pregnancy do not segregate normally grown infants from those who were growth-restricted or dysmature and potentially affected by other causes of IUGR, including chronic hypoxia-acidosis before the onset of labor. Two reports address outcome in prolonged pregnancy newborns with desquamation of skin and wasting of subcutaneous tissue or long, thin bodies. The first study of developmental outcome found an increase in illnesses and sleep disorders, as well as diminished performance on the Vineland Social Maturity Scale. Newborns who were "asphyxiated" before birth had a higher incidence of neurologic signs in the neonatal period (112).

In a second study comparing a similar group of postterm newborns with parchmentlike skin and long, thin bodies with a group of term controls, the postterm group demonstrated lower Brazelton interaction and motor scores than the term controls. By age 8 months, their Bayley motor scores were equivalent, but the mental scores were slightly lower in the postterm group (113). Another report compared the outcome of infants from 129 prolonged pregnancies with the outcome from 184 term control pregnancies. No differences were found with respect to physical milestones or intelligence scores (114).

A 10-year cohort (1978–1987) of term ($n = $ 379,445) and postterm ($n = $ 65,796) births from the Medical Birth Registry of Norway assessed by multivariate analyses provides some indirect insight into the importance of distinguishing the impact of undergrowth and SGA from prolonged pregnancy. The evidence for an adverse impact of postterm birth on perinatal mortality is weak once other factors are taken into account. After controlling for covariates, there was only a slightly increased risk of perinatal mortality in postterm as compared with term births (adjusted RR, 1.11; 95% CI, 0.97–1.27). For postterm births, risk factors for perinatal mortality were SGA (adjusted RR, 5.68; 95% CI, 4.37–7.38) and maternal age 35 years or older (adjusted RR, 1.88; 95% CI, 1.22–2.89), whereas large size for gestational age was a protective factor (adjusted RR, 0.51; 95% CI, 0.26–1.00). Fetal complications were associated with smaller fetal size (115). Unfortunately, because of the nature of the study, no information was provided about the relative impact of fetal malnutrition or postmaturity/dysmaturity in the non-SGA newborn.

Conclusion

- Postterm birth itself appears to be less important than the underlying condition of the infant (eg, SGA) or maternal considerations (eg, maternal age).

References

1. Freud S. Infantile cerebral paralysis. Translated by Lester A. Coral Gables (FL): University of Miami Press; 1968. (Level III)

2. Alberman ED. Cerebral palsy in twins. Guys Hosp Rep 1964;113:285–95. (Level III)

3. Asher P, Schonell FE. A survey of 400 cases of cerebral palsy in childhood. Arch Dis Child 1950;25:360–79. (Level III)

4. Benda CE. Cerebral palsy, birth injuries and anoxia. In: Developmental disorders of mentation and cerebral palsies. New York: Grune & Stratton; 1952. p. 221–91. (Level III)

5. Durkin MV, Kaveggia EG, Pendleton E, Neuhauser G, Opitz JM. Analysis of etiologic factors in cerebral palsy with severe mental retardation. I. Analysis of gestational, parturitional and neonatal data. Eur J Pediatr 1976;123:67–81. (Level II-3)

6. Eastman NJ, Kohl SG, Maisel JE, Kavaler F. The obstetrical background of 753 cases of cerebral palsy. Obstet Gynecol Surv 1962;17:459–500. (Level II-2)

7. Greenspan L, Deaver GG. Clinical approach to the etiology of cerebral palsy. Arch Phys Med Rehabil 1953;34:478–85. (Level III)

8. Illingworth RS, Woods GE. The incidence of twins in cerebral palsy and mental retardation. Arch Dis Child 1960;35:333–5. (Level II-3)

9. Yue SJ. Multiple births in cerebral palsy. Am J Phys Med 1955;34:335–41. (Level III)

10. Russell EM. Cerebral palsied twins. Arch Dis Child 1961;36:328–36. (Level II-2)

11. Steer CM, Bonney W. Obstetric factors in cerebral palsy. Am J Obstet Gynecol 1962;83:526–31. (Level III)

12. Griffiths M. Cerebral palsy in multiple pregnancy. Dev Med Child Neurol 1967;9:713–31. (Level III)

13. Laplaza FJ, Root L, Tassanawipas A, Cervera P. Cerebral palsy in twins. Dev Med Child Neurol 1992;34: 1053–63. (Level III)

14. Grether JK, Nelson KB, Cummins SK. Twinning and cerebral palsy: experience in four northern California counties, births 1983 through 1985. Pediatrics 1993; 92:854–8. (Level II-2)

15. Liu J, Li Z, Lin Q, Zhao P, Zhao F, Hong S, Li S. Cerebral palsy and multiple births in China. Int J Epidemiol 2000;29:292–9. (Level II-2)

16. Nelson KB, Ellenberg JH. Childhood neurological disorders in twins. Paediatr Perinat Epidemiol 1995;9: 135–45. (Level II-2)

17. Petterson B, Nelson KB, Watson L, Stanley F. Twins, triplets, and cerebral palsy in births in Western Australia in the 1980s. BMJ 1993;307:1239–43. (Level II)

18. Pharoah PO, Cooke T. Cerebral palsy and multiple births. Arch Dis Child Fetal Neonatal Ed 1996;75: F174–7. (Level II-2)

19. Williams K, Hennessy E, Alberman E. Cerebral palsy: effects of twinning, birthweight, and gestational age. Arch Dis Child Fetal Neonatal Ed 1996;75: F178– F182. (Level II-2)

20. Yokoyama Y, Shimizu T, Hayakawa K. Prevalence of cerebral palsy in twins, triplets and quadruplets. Int J Epidemiol 1995;24:943–8. (Level II-3)

21. Dunin-Wasowicz D, Rowecka-Trzebicka K, Milewska-Bobula B, Kassur-Siemienska B, Bauer A, Idzik M, et al. Risk factors for cerebral palsy in very low-birth-weight infants in the 1980s and 1990s. J Child Neurol 2000;15:417–20. (Level II-2)

22. Burguet A, Monnet E, Pauchard JY, Roth P, Fromentin C, Dalphin ML, et al. Some risk factors for cerebral palsy in very premature infants: importance of premature rupture of membranes and monochorionic twin placentation. Biol Neonate 1999;75: 177–86. (Level II-2)

23. Minakami H, Honma Y, Matsubara S, Uchida A, Shiraishi H, Sato I. Effects of placental chorionicity on outcome in twin pregnancies. A cohort study. J Reprod Med 1999;44:595–600. (Level II-3)

24. Rydhstroem H. The relationship of birth weight and birth weight discordance to cerebral palsy or mental retardation later in life for twins weighing less than 2500 grams. Am J Obstet Gynecol 1995;173:680–6. (Level II-2)

25. Bejar R, Vigliocco G, Gramajo H, Solana C, Benirschke K, Berry C, et al. Antenatal origin of neurologic damage in newborn infants. II. Multiple gestations. Am J Obstet Gynecol 1990;162:1230–6. (Level II-2)

26. Rydhstroem H, Ingemarsson I. Prognosis and long-term follow-up of a twin after antenatal death of the co-twin. J Reprod Med 1993;38:142–6. (Level II-2)

27. Pharoah PO, Adi Y. Consequences of in-utero death in a twin pregnancy. Lancet 2000;355:1597–602. (Level II-3)

28. Ben-Shlomo I, Alcalay M, Lipitz S, Leibowitz K, Mashiach S, Barkai G. Twin pregnancies complicated

by the death of one fetus. J Reprod Med 1995;40: 458–62. (Level II-2)

29. Eglowstein MS, D'Alton ME. Single intrauterine demise in twin gestation. J Matern Fetal Med 1993;2: 272–5. (Level III)

30. Enbom JA. Twin pregnancy with intrauterine death of one twin. Am J Obstet Gynecol 1985;152:424–9. (Level III)

31. Fusi L, Gordon H. Twin pregnancy complicated by single intrauterine death. Problems and outcomes with conservative management. Br J Obstet Gynaecol 1990;97:511–6. (Level III)

32. Hagay ZJ, Mazor M, Leiberman JR, Biale Y. Management and outcome of multiple pregnancies complicated by the antenatal death of one fetus. J Reprod Med 1986;31:717–20. (Level III)

33. Hanna JH, Hill JM. Single intrauterine fetal demise in multiple gestation. Obstet Gynecol 1984;63:126–30. (Level III)

34. Lumme R, Saarikowski S. Antepartum fetal death of one twin. Int J Gynaecol Obstet 1987;25:331–6. (Level III)

35. Melnick M. Brain damage in survivor after in-utero death of a monozygous co-twin [letter]. Lancet 1977; 2:1287. (Level III)

36. Moore CM, McAdams AJ, Sutherland J. Intrauterine disseminated intravascular coagulation: a syndrome of multiple pregnancy with a dead twin fetus. J Pediatr 1969;74:523–8. (Level III)

37. Petersen IR, Nyholm HC. Multiple pregnancies with single intrauterine demise. Description of twenty-eight pregnancies. Acta Obstet Gynecol Scand 1999;78: 202–6. (Level III)

38. Santema JG, Swaak AM, Wallenberg HC. Expectant management of twin pregnancy with single fetal death. Br J Obstet Gynaecol 1995;102:26–30. (Level II-2)

39. Szymonowicz W, Preston H, Yu VH. The surviving monozygotic twin. Arch Dis Child 1986;61:454–8. (Level III)

40. Wessel J, Schmidt-Gollwitzer K. Intrauterine death of a single fetus in twin pregnancies. J Perinat Med 1988; 16:467–76. (Level III)

41. Yoshiaka H, Kadamoto Y, Mino M, Morikawa Y, Kasubuchi Y, Kusunoki T. Multicystic encephalomalacia in liveborn twin with a stillborn macerated co-twin. J Pediatr 1979;95:798–800. (Level III)

42. Carlson NJ, Towers CV. Multiple gestation complicated by the death of one fetus. Obstet Gynecol 1989; 73:685–9. (Level III)

43. D'Alton ME, Newton ER, Cetrulo CL. Intrauterine fetal demise in multiple gestation. Acta Genet Med Gemellol (Roma) 1984;33:43–9. (Level III)

44. Prompeler HJ, Madjar H, Klosa W, du Bois A, Zahradnik HP, Schillinger H, et al. Twin pregnancies with single fetal death. Acta Obstet Gynecol Scand 1994;73:205–8. (Level III)

45. Van den Veyver IB, Schatteman E, Vanderheyden JS, Van Wiemeersch J, Meulyzer P. Antenatal fetal death in twin pregnancies: a dangerous condition mainly for the surviving co-twin; a report of four cases. Eur J Obstet Gynecol Reprod Biol 1991;38:69–73. (Level III)

46. Van Heteren CF, Nijhuis JG, Semmekrot BA, Mulders LG, van den Berg PP. Risk for surviving twin after fetal death of co-twin in twin-twin transfusion syndrome. Obstet Gynecol 1998;92:215–9. (Level III)

47. Yoshida K, Matayoshi K. A study on the prognosis of surviving cotwin. Acta Genet Med Gemellol (Roma) 1990;39:383–8. (Level III)

48. Kok JH, den Ouden AL, Verloove-Vanhorick SP, Brand R. Outcome of very preterm small for gestational age infants: the first nine years of life. Br J Obstet Gynaecol 1998;105:162–8. (Level II-2)

49. Berg AT. Indices of fetal growth-retardation, perinatal hypoxia-related factors and childhood neurological morbidity. Early Hum Dev 1989;19:271–83. (Level II-2)

50. Montan S, Holmquist P, Ingesson K, Ingemarsson I. Fetal and infant outcome of pregnancies with very early rupture of membranes. Acta Obstet Gynecol Scand 1991;70:119–24. (Level III)

51. Chadwick LM, Pemberton PJ, Kurinczuk JJ. Neonatal subgaleal haematoma: associated risk factors, complications and outcome. J Paediatr Child Health 1996; 32:228–32. (Level II-2)

52. Schatz F. Eine besondere art von einseitiger polyhydramnie mit anderseitiger oligohydramnie bei eineiigen zwillingen. Arch Gynaekol 1882;19:329–69. (German study)

53. Okamura K, Murotsuki J, Tanigawara S, Uehara S, Yajima A. Funipuncture for evaluation of hematologic and coagulation indices in the surviving twin following co-twins death. Obstet Gynecol 1994;83: 975–8. (Level III)

54. Bajoria R. Vascular anatomy of monochorionic placenta in relation to discordant growth and amniotic fluid volume. Hum Reprod 1998;13:2933–40. (Level II-2)

55. Bajoria R. Abundant vascular anastomoses in monoamniotic versus diamniotic monochorionic placentas. Am J Obstet Gynecol 1998;179:788–93. (Level II-2)

56. Dickinson JE, Evans SF. Obstetric and perinatal outcomes from the Australian and New Zealand twin-twin transfusion syndrome registry. Am J Obstet Gynecol 2000;182:706–12. (Level III-3)

57. Fisk NM, Bajoria R, Wigglesworth J. Twin-twin transfusion syndrome. N Engl J Med 1995;333:388; discussion 388–9. (Level III)

58. Hecher K, Plath H, Bregezer T, Hansmann M, Hackeloer BJ. Endoscopic laser surgery versus serial amniocentesis in the treatment of severe twin-twin transfusion syndrome. Am J Obstet Gynecol 1999; 180:717–24. (Level II-2)

59. Johnson JR, Rossi KQ, O'Shaughnessy RW. Amnioreduction versus septostomy in twin-twin transfusion syndrome. Am J Obstet Gynecol 2001; 185:1044–7. (Level II-2)

60. Mari G, Detti L, Oz U, Abuhamad AZ. Long-term outcome in twin-twin transfusion syndrome treated with serial aggressive amnioreduction. Am J Obstst Gynecol 2000;183:211–7. (Level II-3)

61. Mari G, Roberts A, Detti L, Kovanci E, Stefos T, Bahado-Singh RO, et al. Perinatal morbidity and mortality rates in severe twin-twin transfusion syndrome: results of the International Amnioreduction Registry. Am J Obstet Gynecol 2001;185:708–15. (Level II-2)

62. Pinette MG, Pan Y, Pinette SG, Stubblefield PG. Treatment of twin-twin transfusion syndrome. Obstet Gynecol 1993;82:841–6. (Level II-3)

63. Quintero RA, Morales WJ, Allen MH, Bornick PW, Johnson PK, Kruger M. Staging of twin-twin transfusion syndrome. J Perinatol 1999;19:550–5. (Level II-3)

64. Saade GR, Belfort MA, Berry DL, Bui TH, Montgomery LD, Johnson A, et al. Amniotic septostomy for the treatment of twin oligohydramnios-polyhydramnios sequence. Fetal Diagn Ther 1998;13: 86–93. (Level II-3)

65. Saunders NJ, Snijders RJ, Nicolaides KH. Therapeutic amniocentesis in twin-twin transfusion syndrome appearing in the second trimester of pregnancy. Am J Obstet Gynecol 1992;166:820–4. (Level II-3)

66. Fanaroff AA, Martin RJ, Miller MJ. Identification and management of problems in the high-risk neonate. In: Creasy RK, Resnik R, editors. Maternal-fetal medicine. 4th ed. Philadelphia: WB Saunders; 1999. p. 1151–93. (Level III)

67. Alexander GR, Himes JH, Kaufman RB, Mor J, Kogan M. A United States national reference for fetal growth. Obstet Gynecol 1996;87:163–8. (Level II-3)

68. Badawi N, Kurinczuk JJ, Keogh JM, Alessandri LM, O'Sullivan F, Burton PR, et al. Antepartum risk factors for newborn encephalopathy: the Western Australian case-control study. BMJ 1998;317: 1549–53. (Level II-2)

69. McIntire DD, Bloom SL, Casey BM, Leveno KJ. Birth weight in relation to morbidity and mortality among newborn infants. N Engl J Med 1999:340:1234–8. (Level II-2)

70. Goldenberg RL, Nelson KG. Cerebral palsy. In: Creasy RK, Resnik R, editors. Maternal-fetal medicine. 4th ed. Philadelphia: WB Saunders; 1999. p. 1194–1214. (Level III)

71. Brar HS, Rutherford SE. Classification of intrauterine growth retardation. Semin Perinatol 1988;12:2–10. (Level III)

72. Gruenwald P. Chronic fetal distress and placental insufficiency. Biol Neonate 1963;5:215–65. (Level III)

73. Daikoku NH, Johnson JW, Graf C, Kearney K, Tyson JE, King TM. Patterns of intrauterine growth retardation. Obstet Gynecol 1979;54:211–9. (Level II-2)

74. Miller HC, Hassanein K. Diagnosis of impaired fetal growth in newborn infants. Pediatrics 1971;48: 511–22. (Level II-3)

75. Villar J, de Onis M, Kestler E, Bolaros F, Cerezo R, Berredes H. The differential neonatal morbidity of the intrauterine growth retardation syndrome. Am J Obstet Gynecol 1990;163:151–7. (Level II-2)

76. Chard T, Yoong A, Macintosh M. The myth of fetal growth retardation at term. Br J Obstet Gynaecol 1993;100:1076–81. (Level III)

77. Low JA, Galbraith RS, Muir D, Killen H, Pater B, Karchmar J. Intrauterine growth retardation: a study of long-term morbidity. Am J Obstet Gynecol 1982; 142:670–7. (Level II-2)

78. Uvebrant P, Hagberg G. Intrauterine growth in children with cerebral palsy. Acta Paediatr 1992;81: 407–12. (Level II-2)

79. Gilles FH, Leviton A, Dooling EC. The developing human brain: growth and epidemiologic neuropathology. Boston (MA): John Wright; 1983. (Level III)

80. Sims ME, Turkel SB, Halterman G, Paul RH. Brain injury and intrauterine death. Am J Obstet Gynecol 1985;151:721–3. (Level III)

81. Gaffney G, Sellers S, Flavell V, Johnson A, Squier M, Johnson A. Case-control study of intrapartum care, cerebral palsy, and perinatal death. BMJ 1994;308: 743–50. (Level II-2)

82. Low JA, Handley-Derry MH, Burke SO, Peters RD, Pater EA, Killen HL, et al. Association of intrauterine fetal growth retardation and learning deficits at age 9 to 11 years. Am J Obstet Gynecol 1992;167: 1499–1505. (Level II-3)

83. Blair E, Stanley F. Intrauterine growth and spastic cerebral palsy. I. Association with birth weight for gestational age. Am J Obstet Gynecol 1990;162:229–37. (Level II-2)

84. Blair E, Stanley F. Intrauterine growth and spastic cerebral palsy. II. The association with morphology at birth. Early Hum Dev 1992;28:91–103. (Level II-2)

85. Barker DJ, editor. Fetal and infant origins of adult disease: papers written by the Medical Research Council Environmental Epidemiology Unit, University of Southampton. London: British Medical Journal; 1992. (Level III)

86. Veelken N, Stollhoff K, Claussen M. Development and perinatal risk factors of very low-birth-weight infants. Small versus appropriate for gestational age. Neuropediatrics 1992;23:102–7. (Level II-2)

87. Murphy DJ, Sellers S, Mac Kenzie IZ, Yudkin PL, Johnson A. Case-control study of antenatal and intrapartum risk factors for cerebral palsy in very preterm singleton babies. Lancet 1995;346:1449–54. (Level II-2)

88. Nelson KB, Grether JK. Can magnesium sulfate reduce the risk of cerebral palsy in very low birth-weight infants? Pediatrics 1995;95:263–9. (Level II-2)

89. Mittendorf R, Dambrosia J, Pryde PG, Lee KS, Gianopoulos JG, Besinger RE, et al. Association between the use of antenatal magnesium sulfate in preterm labor and adverse health outcomes in infants. Am J Obstet Gynecol 2002;186:1111–8. (Level I)

90. Grether JK, Hoogstrate J, Walsh-Greene E, Nelson KB. Magnesium sulfate for tocolysis and risk of spastic cerebral palsy in premature children born to women without preeclampsia. Am J Obstet Gynecol 2000;183:717–25. (Level II-2)

91. Antonov AN. Children born during the siege of Leningrad in 1942. J Pediatr 1947;30:250–9. (Level III)

92. Smith CA. Effects of maternal undernutrition upon the newborn infant in Holland (1944-1945). J Pediatr 1947;30:229–43. (Level III)

93. Nathan L, Leveno KJ, Carmody TJ, Kelly MA, Sherman ML. Meconium: a 1990s perspective on an old obstetric hazard. Obstet Gynecol 1994;83: 329–32. (Level II-2)

94. Jazayeri A, Politz L, Tsibris JC, Queen T, Spellacy WN. Fetal erythropoietin levels in pregnancies complicated by meconium passage: does meconium suggest fetal hypoxia? Am J Obstet Gynecol 2000;183: 188–90. (Level II-2)

95. Yeomans ER, Gilstrap LC 3d, Leveno KJ, Burris JS. Meconium in the amniotic fluid and fetal acid-based status. Obstet Gynecol 1989;73:175–8. (Level II-3)

96. Dijxhoorn MJ, Visser GH, Fidler VJ, Touwen BC, Huisjes HJ. Apgar score, meconium and acidaemia at birth in relation to neonatal neurological morbidity in term infants. Br J Obstet Gynaecol 1986;93:217–22. (Level II-2)

97. Nelson KB, Ellenberg JH. Obstetric complications as risk factors for cerebral palsy or seizure disorder. JAMA 1984;251:1843–8. (Level II-2)

98. Nelson KB, Grether JK. Potentially asphyxiating conditions and spastic cerebral palsy in infants of normal birth weight. Am J Obstet Gynecol 1998;179:507–13. (Level II-2)

99. Altshuler G, Hyde S. Meconium-induced vasocontraction: a potential cause of cerebral and other fetal hypoperfusion and of poor pregnancy outcome. J Child Neurol 1989;4:137–42. (Level III)

100. Kafkasli A, Belfort MA, Giannina G, Vedernikov YP, Schaffner DL, Popek EJ. Histopathologic effects of meconium on human umbilical artery and vein: in vitro study. J Matern Fetal Med 1997;6:356–61. (Level II-2)

101. Sienko A, Altshuler G. Meconium-induced umbilical vascular necrosis in abortuses and fetuses; a histopathologic study for cytokines. Obstet Gynecol 1999;94:415–20. (Level III)

102. Montgomery LD, Belfort MA, Saade GR, Moise KJ Jr, Vedernikov YP. Meconium inhibits the contraction of umbilical vessels induced by the thromboxane A 2 analog U 46619. Am J Obstet Gynecol 1995;173: 1075–8. (Level II-2)

103. Hankins GD, Rowe J, Quirk JG Jr, Trubey R, Strickland DM. Significance of brown and/or green amniotic fluid at the time of second trimester genetic amniocentesis. Obstet Gynecol 1984;64:353–8. (Level II-2)

104. Mazor M, Froimovich M, Lazer S, Maymon E, Glezerman M. Listeria monocytogenes. The role of transabdominal amniocentesis in febrile patients with preterm labor. Arch Gynecol Obstet 1992;252: 109–12. (Level III)

105. Valkenburg MH, Essed GG, Potters HV. Perinatal listerosis underdiagnosed as a cause of preterm labor? Eur J Obstet Gynecol Reprod Biol 1988;27:283–8. (Level III)

106. Romero R, Hanaoka S, Mazor M, Athanassiadis AP, Callahan R, Hsu YC, et al. Meconium-stained amniotic fluid: a risk factor for microbial invasion of the amniotic cavity. Am J Obstet Gynecol 1991;164: 859–62. (Level II-2)

107. Agency for Healthcare Research and Quality. Management of prolonged pregnancy. Evidence Report/ Technical Assessment 53. Rockville (MD): AHRQ; 2002. Publication no. 02-E018. (Level III)

108. Zwerdling, MA. Factors pertaining to prolonged pregnancy and its outcome. Pediatrics 1967;40:202–12. (Level II-2)

109. Pollack RN, Hauer-Pollack G, Divon MY. Macrosomia in postdates pregnancy: the accuracy of routine ultrasonographic screening. Am J Obstet Gynecol 1992;167:7–11. (Level II-2)

110. Boyd ME, Usher RH, McLean FH, Kramer MS. Obstetric consequences of postmaturity. Am J Obstet Gynecol 1988;158:334–8. (Level II-2)

111. Kramer MS, McLean FH, Boyd ME, Usher RH. The validity of gestational age estimation by menstrual dating in term, preterm, and postterm gestations. JAMA 1988;260:3306–8. (Level II-2)

112. Lovell KE. The effect of postmaturity on the developing child. Med J Aust 1973;1:13–7. (Level II-2)

113. Field TM, Dabiri C, Hallock N, Schuman HH. Developmental effects of prolonged pregnancy and the postmaturity syndrome. J Pediatr 1977;90:836–9. (Level II-2)

114. Shime J, Librach CL, Gare DJ, Cook CJ. The influence of prolonged pregnancy on infant development at one and two years of age: a prospective controlled study. Am J Obstet Gynecol 1986;154:341–5. (Level II-1)

115. Campbell MK, Ostbye T, Ergens LM. Post-term birth: risk factors and outcomes in a 10-year cohort of Norwegian births. Obstet Gynecol 1997;89:543–8. (Level II-2)

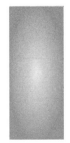

CHAPTER 5

NEONATAL ASSESSMENT

Evaluation of the Term or Near-Term Infant with Encephalopathy

Encephalopathy in the term or near-term newborn infant is manifested by serious neurologic depression in the delivery room and nursery. Clinical signs observable in the delivery room include low Apgar score and its components and correlates, such as hypotonia; depressed reflexes including cry, suck, absent Moro's reflex; decreased consciousness; difficulty in initiating and maintaining respiration; poor color; and bradycardia.

Assessment of the depressed neonate should be guided by the differential diagnosis, with the aim of understanding etiology and identifying conditions for which treatment is feasible. Major intrapartum events capable of interrupting oxygen supply to the fetus, such as abruption of the placenta, umbilical cord prolapse, or uterine rupture, especially if accompanied by prolonged bradycardia, may suggest hypoxia–ischemia as a cause. However, no interventions have been shown to benefit the infant with hypoxic–ischemic encephalopathy (HIE) (1), and even when there is a clearcut obstetric complication, it is important to explore other diagnostic possibilities for which treatment might improve the ultimate outcome.

In the delivery room, birth of a seriously depressed infant should lead to an immediate effort to gather information helpful in understanding etiology, especially after an uncomplicated delivery. An examination of the umbilical cord, membranes, and placenta may assist in the clinical–pathologic correlation when there is an adverse perinatal outcome. Samples should be drawn to determine arterial cord pH and base deficit levels. Following rapid assessment of the adequacy of the resuscitation, the clinician should reglove, split the amnion from the chorion, and take a culture sample from between the membranes. Other culture samples, although less informative in the presence of prolonged rupture of membranes, may be worthwhile.

The mother's history should be examined, and maternal and family medical conditions, including thyroid or other autoimmune disorders, deep vein and other thrombotic disorders, intolerance to oral contraceptives, early stroke or myocardial infarction, and history of prior pregnancy loss, should be considered. The history should evaluate whether a twin fetus died, even early in the pregnancy. A history of maternal infection should be sought, including clinical markers of chorioamnionitis or sexually transmitted disease. The history also should look for evidence of intrapartum maternal fever.

In the past, it had been common to diagnose HIE in the neonate unless major malformation, culture-proven sepsis, drug overdose, or serious metabolic defect was recognized. It is now clear that the differential diagnosis is considerably larger. Further, identification of one risk factor does not rule out the presence of other and interacting determinants of risk. Multiple risk factors can substantially augment risk; among symptomatic infants, it is not unusual to find more than a single factor contributing to adverse outcome.

The newborn should be evaluated for infection with appropriate blood cultures. There is increasing information on the value of C-reactive protein as an indicator of an inflammatory response, and in the future, there is likely to be value in the measurement of inflammatory mediators such as cytokines and chemokines in the clinical setting.

Examining indicators of thrombophilia, such as antiphospholipid antibodies, the factor V Leiden mutation, protein-C and protein-S levels, and prothrombin gene deletions, should be considered for the mother and infant if there are persistent signs of thrombosis or stroke.

Apgar Score

The Apgar score is a standardized mini-examination of brainstem function assessing the clinical status of the newborn in the first minutes after birth (2, 3). There are numerous factors that can affect the Apgar score. These include preterm birth, maternal sedation or anesthesia, congenital malformations, and the individual assigning the score (4). Cardiorespiratory conditions also may decrease the newborn's heart rate, respiration, and tone. Infection may interfere with tone, color, and response to resuscitative efforts, and additional information is required to interpret Apgar scores properly in infants receiving resuscitation. Thus, to attribute a low Apgar score solely to asphyxia or hypoxia represents a misuse of the score.

A 5-minute Apgar score of 7–10 is considered "normal." Scores of 4, 5, and 6 are intermediate and are not markers of high levels of risk of later neurologic dysfunction. A low Apgar score (<4) is a nonspecific indicator of illness in the neonate and often is the first recognizable marker of encephalopathy. However, a low 1- or 5-minute score alone does not demonstrate that later development of cerebral palsy was caused by perinatal asphyxia, and it is well established that the 1- or 5-minute Apgar score is a poor predictor of long-term neurologic outcome in the individual patient (5). Even a 5-minute score of 0–3, although possibly a result of hypoxia, is limited as an indicator of the severity of the problem and correlates poorly with future neurologic outcome (5, 6). An Apgar score of 0–3 at 5 minutes is associated with an increased risk of cerebral palsy in term infants of only 0.3–1% (5, 6). Almost 90% of infants with 10-minute Apgar scores of 0–3 did not have subsequent cerebral palsy (5). Conversely, 75% of children with cerebral palsy had normal Apgar scores at birth (5). The 5-minute Apgar score, and particularly the change or lack of change in the score between 1 and 5 minutes, reflects both prenatal events as well as the effectiveness of the resuscitation efforts (7).

In spite of established data to the contrary, low Apgar scores were used as the primary criteria for defining birth asphyxia by the ninth revision of the International Classification of Diseases ICD-9 coding system. This led the American College of Obstetricians and Gynecologists (ACOG) and the American Academy of Pediatrics to establish two documents on the subject: "Use and Misuse of the Apgar Score" (published in 1986) and "Use and Abuse of the Apgar Score" (published in 1996). The first joint statement was reaffirmed in 1989 and 1991 and replaced by the 1996 joint statement. The 1996 joint statement updates the former and was reaffirmed in 1997 and 1999 (8). This Task Force continues to support these documents. It should be noted that a recent retrospective cohort analysis (151,891 live-born singleton infants without malformations delivered at 26 weeks of gestation or later) concluded that the 5-minute Apgar score continues to be a valid predictor of neonatal survival in large populations (9). However, the same study also found that it is inappropriate to use the Apgar score to predict long-term neurologic outcome.

Studies have demonstrated a good correlation between extremely low Apgar scores (<3) and neurologic disability. A score of less than 3 at 15 minutes was associated with a 53% mortality rate and a 36% cerebral palsy rate. When a low score persisted at 20 minutes, mortality was almost 60% and more than one half (57%) had cerebral palsy (5). However, even with extremely low (<3) scores there is potential for some improvement at 10, 15, and 20 minutes after birth. For example, 17% of newborns with 10-minute scores of less than 3 had cerebral palsy, but the rate dropped to approximately 5% if the score improved at 15 and 20 minutes (5). The risk of poor neurologic outcome increases when the Apgar score remains less than 4 at 10, 15, and 20 minutes (5, 10). Table 5–1 indicates the relative risk of death and disability stratified according to the 5-minute Apgar score (11). On the basis of all of the previously described studies, the Task Force supports ACOG's position that an Apgar score of 0–3 after 5 minutes remains an appropriate criteria for use as a potential marker of intrapartum asphyxia.

The Role of Neuroimaging in Defining the Timing and Severity of Neonatal Encephalopathy and Cerebral Palsy

Several patterns of brain injury may result from hypoxic–ischemic episodes in the fetus and depend on the severity of the cerebral hypotension, the maturity of the brain at the time of injury, and the duration or recurrence of the event (12). These variables preclude absolute precision in the timing of the injury by neuroimaging.

When blood flow to the brain is mildly or moderately reduced, blood is shunted from the anterior to the posterior circulation to maintain adequate perfusion to the brain stem, cerebellum, and basal ganglia. However, when reduction of cerebral blood flow is severe, autoregulation is impaired, and the deep structures of the brain are involved (13).

When these events occur in the preterm fetus, injury typically occurs in the periventricular white matter, with sparing of the subcortical white matter and cerebral cortex (12). In contrast, term infants sustain injury in the "watershed" portions of the cerebral cortex and its underlying subcortical and periventricular white

Table 5–1. Relative Risk of Death and Disabilities According to 5-Minute Apgar Score*

Outcome	Relative Risk (95% confidence interval)	
	Apgar Score 0–3	Apgar Score 4–6
Death		
Neonatal	386 (270–552)	45 (30–68)
Infant	76 (56–103)	8.9 (6.4–12)
Age 1–8 y	18 (8.5–39)	2.2 (0.9–5.4)
Disability		
Cerebral palsy	81 (48–138)	31 (22–44)
Mental retardation without cerebral palsy	9.4 (3–29)	4.4 (2.2–8.8)
Neurologic disabilities without cerebral palsy or mental retardation	8.8 (4.7–17)	2.1 (1.2–3.6)
Non-neurologic disabilities	1.7 (0.8–3.5)	1.3 (0.9–1.8)

*Relative risks were approximated by odds ratios in logistic regression models. The category of 5-minute Apgar scores 7–10 was used as a reference.
Modified from Moster D, Lie RT, Irgens LM, Bjerkedal T, Markestad T. The association of Apgar score with subsequent death and cerebral palsy: a population-based study in term infants. J Pediatr 2001;138:798–803.

matter. Consequently, periventricular white matter damage (eg, periventricular leukomalacia) is a common finding in preterm fetuses with cerebral palsy. In contrast, between 34–36 weeks of gestation, the pattern of injury begins to change, and the regions of the brain at highest risk include the subcortical white matter and cerebral cortex. After 36 weeks gestation, prominent activity is noted almost entirely in these high-risk areas when an insult occurs. (12).

Preterm Infants

In the acute phase after an ischemic injury in the preterm infant, transcranial ultrasonography may show ventricular compression and mildly increased echogenicity secondary to edema. These findings are not reliable, however, as small ventricles can be normal, and apparently increased echogenicity can be the result of improper power or gain settings on the ultrasound machine. The two most common locations for periventricular leukomalacia are the posterior periventricular white matter adjacent to the lateral aspect of the trigone of the lateral ventricles and the white matter adjacent to the foramina of Monro. The best early ultrasonographic sign of periventricular white-matter injury is the periventricular "flare" (the loss of the normal regularly spaced parenchymal echoes) and increased echogenicity (14). However, a definitive diagnosis of periventricular leukomalacia by ultrasonogram requires the demonstration of cavitation (15). This occurs between 10 days and 6 weeks after the ischemic episode (but usually at <3 weeks).

Computed tomography (CT) and magnetic resonance imaging (MRI) do not play a major role in the early diagnosis of periventricular leukomalacia because of the difficulty involved in transporting and caring for sick preterm neonates. However, MRI and CT are useful for the diagnosis of end-stage periventricular leukomalacia in later infancy and childhood and also may be useful in diagnosing mild cases of periventricular leukomalacia when nonspecific ventriculomegaly is the only detectable abnormality on ultrasonography.

In the preterm infant who has sustained severe cerebral hypoperfusion during fetal life, injury is predominantly in the deep gray matter and brain stem nuclei. Ultrasonography in the first 2 days after birth may be normal, but by the second or third day, hyperechogenicity may be detected in the basal ganglia and thalami. Computed tomography will show hypodensity of the thalami and basal ganglia, while MRI studies acquired in the first 2 days after injury will show reduced diffusion and elevated lactate (12).

The preterm infant also may sustain germinal matrix and intraventricular hemorrhage, the severity and grading of which may be evaluated by ultrasonography. Germinal matrix hemorrhage may be observed and is characterized as a region of increased echogenicity. The intraventricular hemorrhage results in filling a portion of or sometimes all of the ventricular system with echogenic material. In the first few weeks after the acute event, the intraventricular clot organizes and becomes well-defined and less echogenic. Hemorrhage also can be detected by CT; it appears hyperdense in the acute phase and becomes isodense at 7–10 days after the bleed. Temporal evolution of intraventricular blood in neonates has not been studied by MRI (12).

Term Infants

Severe, acute hypoxic and hypotensive insult results in injury in the deeper brain substance, including the lateral thalami, posterior putamina, hippocampi, and corticospinal tracts (16). These injuries result in athetosis, quadriparesis, severe seizure disorders, and mental retardation. Standard imaging studies are typically normal if performed on the day of birth. However, MRI spectroscopy will show an increase in lactate within hours of injury (17, 18). Diffusion-weighted imaging will show reduced water motion within the first 24 hours after onset of injury and has better resolution than ultrasound (19, 20); the abnormal diffusion peaks by about 5 days and disappears within 2 weeks (20).

Ultrasonography, CT, and MRI reveal specific findings over a period of days to weeks that may be of help in determining the timing and severity of the injury, as well as the prognosis (see Table 5–2). Ultrasonography shows increased thalamic and basal ganglia echogenicity by 2–3 days after injury. Computed tomography shows low attenuation of the thalami by about 24 hours after injury (21). Standard MRI sequences show absence of the normal high T1 in the posterior limb of the internal capsule by about 24 hours. Abnormal high signal appears in the lateral thalami and posterior lentiform nuclei by the third day after injury (22). This high signal then coalesces into a smaller focus in the lateral thalamus and posterior putamen, where it remains visible for 2–4 months (12). High T2 signal appears in these areas by the end of the second week and may remain for decades (16).

Conclusion

- Although neuroimaging techniques can be helpful in the timing of an injury, they can only approximate a window in time rather than determine the moment when injury occurred with absolute precision.

Neonatal Electroencephalography

The neonatal electroencephalography examination is a widely available, inexpensive, and noninvasive neurologic test of the functional integrity of the newborn brain. The prognostic value of neonatal electroencephalography examinations is well recognized. If, at the height of an illness, the background shows marked abnormalities (eg, burst suppression, isoelectricity, or extremely low voltage), there is a reasonable expectation for a high risk of death or subsequent chronic static encephalopathy in the survivors (23–26). If the electroencephalogram recording were normal or only mildly abnormal, a favorable outcome can be anticipated (27).

Table 5–2. Summary of Imaging Findings in Relation to the Time of Birth Injury*

Modality	Finding	Timing
Proton MRI spectroscopy	Increased lactate	Onset in first few hours, lasts about 2 weeks
	Decreased N-acetyl aspartate	Onset in first few hours, persists indefinitely
Diffusion MRI	Reduced diffusion	Onset in <24 hours, normalizes in 7–10 days
	Increased diffusion	Onset in 10–15 days, persists indefinitely
T1-weighted MRI	Increased signal in thalamus or basal ganglia	Onset at 2–3 days, persists for months, becoming more localized and globular
	Loss of signal in posterior limb of internal capsule	Onset in <24 hours
T2-weighted MRI	Increased signal in cortex or deep nuclei	Onset in <24 hours, persists several days
	Decreased signal	Onset at 6–7 days, persists for months
CT scan	Decreased density in thalami or basal ganglia	Onset in <24 hours, persists for 5–7 days
Ultrasonography	Increased echogenicity in thalami or basal ganglia	Onset at approximately 24 hours, progresses over 2–3 days, persists for 5–7 days

Abbreviations: CT, computed tomography; MRI, magnetic resonance imaging.

*These times are only approximate and can vary with the severity and duration of the injury. There also is some patient-to-patient variability.

Data from Barkovich AJ, Baranski K, Vigneron D, Partridge JC, Hallam DK, Hajnal BL, et al. Proton MR spectroscopy for the evaluation of brain injury in asphyxiated, term neonates. AJNR Am J Neuroradiol 1999;20:1399–405; Barkovich AJ, Hallam D. Neuroimaging in perinatal hypoxic-ischemic injury. Ment Retard Dev Disabil Res Rev 1997;3:28–41; Barkovich AJ, Westmark K, Ferriero DM, Partridge C, Sola A. Perinatal asphyxia: MR findings in the first 10 days. AJNR Am J Neuroradiol 1995;16:427–38; Barkovich AJ. MR and CT evaluation of profound neonatal and infantile asphyxia. AJNR Am J Neuroradiol 1992;13:959–72; discussion 973–5; and Roland EH, Poskitt K, Rodriguez E, Lupton BA, Hill A. Perinatal hypoxic-ischemic thalamic injury: clinical features and neuroimaging. Ann Neurol 1998;44:161–66.

The specificity of the electroencephalography examination is very limited. In acute causes of global encephalopathy (eg, perinatal asphyxia, shock, meningitis, or hypoglycemia), there are no distinctive kinds of diffuse electroencephalography abnormalities that uniquely reveal the cause of the encephalopathy. An abnormal neonatal electroencephalography examination only reveals how potently the abnormality has disturbed brain function. Likewise, for acute causes of focal encephalopathy (eg, localized stroke or hemorrhage), the electroencephalography may reveal the magnitude of the disturbance (the abundance of focal slowing, seizures, or excessive sharp waves) but does not reveal the identity of the cause.

Scant attention has been paid to the use of neonatal electroencephalography in determining the timing of the onset of an acute encephalopathy. There is such great individual patient variation in the type, evolution, and severity of electroencephalography abnormalities observed in acute encephalopathies that the question of timing will not be answered by electroencephalography alone.

Conclusions

- Electroencephalography may provide early evidence of the presence and severity of encephalopathy.

- Electroencephalography is the premier tool for identifying neonatal seizures and distinguishing them from other phenomena.

- Electroencephalography does not indicate the cause of encephalopathy.

- A normal electroencephalography in the first 7 days after birth is evidence against an acute intrapartum injury.

Placental Pathology Related to Neonatal Encephalopathy and Cerebral Palsy

Numerous placental pathologic findings have been described in children who subsequently developed cerebral palsy. However, there are too few properly designed studies to identify a cause-and-effect relationship between any specific lesion and the development of cerebral palsy.

For example, it is now clear that intrauterine infection is a risk factor for subsequent development of cerebral palsy (also see Chapter 2) (28–30). Clinical chorioamnionitis has a relative risk (RR) of 4.7 (95% confidence interval [CI], 1.3–16.2) for development of cerebral palsy among term infants and 1.9 (95% CI, 1.4–2.5) among preterm infants. Histologic chorioamnionitis had a RR of 1.6 for preterm infants, but the CI included 1 (95% CI, 0.9–2.9) (31). However, the resulting placental pathology may only represent an associated finding of the ongoing infectious process, rather than a cause and effect. The significance of other findings, such as villous edema, hemorrhagic endovasculitis, and chronic villitis has not been well delineated, and disagreement persists as to the underlying resulting pathophysiology or even the consistency of clinical correlations with these findings.

Reports that suggest thrombosis within large fetal vessels in the placenta may be related to HIE and cerebral palsy merit further study, but conclusions should not be drawn regarding the timing of the brain insult, nor do they necessarily delineate a specific underlying disease process (32–35).

The twin-to-twin transfusion syndrome, associated with a monochorionic placentation and death of a co-twin, is a significant risk factor for cerebral palsy. The pathogenesis and timing of the injury requires additional investigation (36).

Detailed examination of the placenta is always potentially informative, but further research is required to more accurately define the role of specific placental lesions in the development of fetal or neonatal brain injury.

Conclusions

- Placental pathology may be useful in suggesting an infectious cause when signs of chorioamnionitis are present and the neonate has encephalopathy.

- Placental pathology is essential in determining chorionicity in multiple gestation pregnancies

Nucleated Red Blood Cells and Lymphocyte Counts and Neurologic Impairment

Neonatal nucleated red blood cells are immature erythrocytes whose significance in term newborns is unclear and somewhat controversial (37). Some investigators have reported an association between the number of nucleated red blood cells and intrauterine hypoxia or asphyxia (37, 38), supporting earlier findings that nucleated red blood cell counts were useful in the timing of fetal neurologic injury (39, 40). Other studies have reported an increase in both lymphocyte and nucleated red blood cell counts in term infants with HIE and permanent neurologic impairment (41). Further, an association between elevated lymphocyte and normoblast counts and "brain-damaging ischemia and hypoxia" has been reported (42). However, a more recent study reported that the use of lymphocyte counts was less useful because of "rapid normalization" in the first few hours after birth (41).

One study compared 441 preterm infants to determine if there was a difference in nucleated red blood cell counts between infants who developed periventricular leukomalacia and intraventricular hemorrhage and those who did not. No significant difference was reported (44). However, another study of 359 preterm infants did report an increase in neonatal nucleated red blood cells in association with histologic chorioamnionitis. Those authors proposed that the erythropoietic response in the fetus might be caused by either inflammation or increased erythropoietin (44).

Other potential markers of perinatal or intrauterine hypoxia that have been studied include erythropoietin, creatine phosphokinase, hypoxanthine, and arginine vasopressin levels (45–48). The clinical utility of these markers for the prediction, etiology, or timing of neurologic insult remains to be determined.

Conclusion

- Although nucleated red blood cells and lymphocytes may be elevated in some newborns with neonatal encephalopathy and subsequent neurologic dysfunction, the clinical utility of these measurements to determine the timing of neurologic injury should be considered investigational.

Focal Ischemic Stroke as a Mechanism of Cerebral Injury in the Perinatal Period

Cerebral infarction may affect 1 in 4,000 live term births, and more than 50% of infants with perinatal infarction may develop cerebral palsy, with hemiplegic cerebral palsy being the most common subtype (49–51). At least 20% of children with hemiplegic cerebral palsy have radiologic evidence of infarction in the prenatal or perinatal period (52, 53). Focal arterial ischemic stroke usually is caused by arterial thrombosis or embolism from fetal vessels or from the placenta. In an autopsy series of almost 600 infants, 5% had evidence of cerebral infarcts, with embolization being the most common cause. Perinatal stroke also may be caused by decreased blood pressure or oxygenation leading to vascular injury (54) or trauma to major arteries (55).

Evidence of neonatal arterial ischemic stroke often is recognized as a result of neuroimaging undertaken because the neonate has seizures during the first few days after birth (56–59). Some seizures may be subtle and easily missed (60). Infants also may present with apnea, lethargy, or hypotonia (56). It is rare for signs of a hemiparesis to be recognized before age 6 months (52, 61). A recent study has described a series of children who appeared normal in the neonatal period but presented with pathologic early hand preference or seizures at older than 2 months, leading to the diagnosis of what is presumed to be prenatal or perinatal infarct (62). Sinovenous thrombosis is the formation of clots in the cerebral veins or venous sinuses. Impaired venous drainage of cerebral blood flow leads to cerebral edema, which may progress to unilateral or bilateral infarction (51, 63).

The causes of neonatal cerebral infarction are not usually clear. One study reported unknown etiology in 52% of cases. Asphyxia was felt to be contributory in 33%; postnatal hypotension, meningitis, coagulopathies, polycythemia, and hypernatremia each accounted for 2%; and cocaine exposure and congenital heart disease each accounted for 1% (63). In an autopsy case series, disseminated intravascular coagulopathy or sepsis or both were felt to be contributory in 20 of 29 cases studied (64).

Both preeclampsia, which can be related to coagulation disorders, and maternal infection may predispose the fetus to perinatal infarction in the neonate by causing placental vasculopathy and hypoperfusion. Preeclampsia may cause atherosis of the placental vascular bed, and chorioamnionitis may lead to both vasculitis and vasoconstriction (65). Atherosis, vasculitis, and vasoconstriction may all lead to thrombosis with subsequent embolization. The patent foramen ovale present in the fetus and newborn may allow emboli that enter the systemic venous circulation to reach the cerebral arterial circulation. Impairment of placental blood flow also may lead to fetal hypoxemia.

Multiple perinatal risk factors, including thrombophilic disorders, maternal–fetal transfusion, congenital heart disease, and trauma (50, 66–70), may act simultaneously to cause fetal or neonatal cerebral infarction. A study has reported abnormal levels of both coagulation and inflammatory factors in neonatal blood samples from children with cerebral palsy, suggesting both may contribute to abnormal thrombosis in the perinatal period (28). The period of risk does not end with delivery. Infants who acquire maternally transmitted infections during delivery or other infections in the nursery may develop meningitis and go on to have infarctions from the resulting vasculitis (71).

Conclusions

- Hemiplegic cerebral palsy is not associated with global intrapartum hypoxia; however, perinatal strokes are a cause of cerebral palsy, particularly hemiplegic cerebral palsy.

- Maternal infection, prothrombic disorders in the mother or infant or both, congenital heart disease in the infant, maternal–fetal

transfusion, trauma during delivery, and neonatal sepsis and dehydration may all play a role in the etiology of perinatal stroke.

References

1. Whitelaw A. Systematic review of therapy after hypoxic-ischaemic brain injury in the perinatal period. Semin Neonatol 2000;5:33–40. (Level III)

2. Apgar V. A proposal for a new method of evaluation of the newborn infant. Curr Res Anesth Analg 1953; 32:260–7. (Level III)

3. Apgar V, Holaday DA, James LS, Weisbrot IM, Berrien C. Evaluation of the newborn infant: second report. JAMA 1958;168:1985–8. (Level III)

4. Ramin SM, Gilstrap LC 3rd, Leveno KJ, Burris JC, Little BB. Umbilical artery acid-base status in the preterm infant. Obstet Gynecol 1989;74:256–8. (Level II-2)

5. Nelson KB, Ellenberg JH. Apgar score as predictors of chronic neurologic disability. Pediatrics 1981;68: 36–44. (Level II-2)

6. Stanley FJ. Cerebral palsy trends: implications for perinatal care. Acta Obstet Gynecol Scand 1994;73L: 5–9. (Level III)

7. Perlman JM, Risser R. Cardiopulmonary resuscitation in the delivery room. Associated clinical events. Arch Pediatr Adolesc Med 1995;149:20–5. (Level II-2)

8. American Academy of Pediatrics, American College of Obstetricians and Gynecologists. Use and abuse of the Apgar score. ACOG Committee Opinion 174. Elk Grove Village (IL): AAP; Washington, DC: ACOG; 1996. (Level III)

9. Casey BM, McIntire DD, Leveno KJ. The continuing value of the Apgar score for the assessment of newborn infants. N Engl J Med 2001;344:467–71. (Level II-2)

10. Freeman JM, Nelson KB. Intrapartum asphyxia and cerebral palsy. Pediatrics 1988;82:240–9. (Level III)

11. Moster D, Lie RT, Irgens LM, Bjerkedal T, Markestad T. The association of Apgar score with subsequent death and cerebral palsy: a population-based study in term infants. J Pediatr 2001;138:798–803. (Level II-2)

12. Barkovich AJ, Hallam D. Neuroimaging in perinatal hypoxic-ischemic injury. Ment Retard Dev Disabil Res Rev 1997;3:28–41. (Level III)

13. Ashwal S, Majcher JS, Longo DL. Patterns of fetal lamb regional cerebral blood flow during and after prolonged hypoxia: studies during the posthypoxic recovery period. Am J Obstet Gynecol 1981;139: 365–72. (Animal study)

14. Baarsma R, Laurini RN, Baerts W, Okken A. Reliability of sonography in non-hemorrhagic periventricular leucomalacia. Pediatr Radiol 1987;17: 189–91. (Level III)

15. Dubowitz LM, Bydder GM, Mushin J. Developmental sequence of periventricular leukomalacia. Correlation of ultrasound clinical, and nuclear magnetic resonance functions. Arch Dis Child 1985;60:349–55. (Level III)

16. Barkovich AJ. MR and CT evaluation of profound neonatal and infantile asphyxia. AJNR Am J Neuroradiol 1992;13:959–72; discussion 973–5. (Level III)

17. Amess PN, Penrice J, Wylezinska M, Lorek A, Townsend J, Wyatt JS, et al. Early brain proton magnetic resonance spectroscopy and neonatal neurology related to neurodevelopmental outcome at 1 year in term infants after presumed hypoxic-ischaemic brain injury. Dev Med Child Neurol 1999;41:436–45. (Level II-2)

18. Hanrahan JD, Cox IJ, Azzopardi D, Cowan FM, Sargentoni J, Bell JD, et al. Relation between proton magnetic resonance spectroscopy within 18 hours of birth asphyxia and neurodevelopment at 1 year of age. Dev Med Child Neurol 1999;41:76–82. (Level II-2)

19. Cowan FM, Pennock JM, Hanrahan JD, Manji KP, Edwards AD. Early detection of cerebral infarction and hypoxic ischemic encephalopathy in neonates using diffusion-weighted magnetic resonance imaging. Neuropediatrics 1994;25:172–5. (Level III)

20. Robertson RL, Ben-Sira L, Barnes PD, Mulkern RV, Robson CD, Maier SE, et al. MR line-scan diffusion-weighted imaging of term neonates with perinatal brain ischemia. AJNR Am J Neuroradiol 1999;20:1658–70. (Level II-3)

21. Roland EH, Poskitt K, Rodriguez E, Lupton BA, Hill A. Perinatal hypoxic-ischemic thalamic injury: clinical features and neuroimaging. Ann Neurol 1998;44:161–6. (Level III)

22. Barkovich AJ, Westmark KD, Ferriero DM, Sola A, Partridge JC. Perinatal asphyxia: MR findings in the first 10 days. AJNR Am J Neuroradiol 1995;16:427–38. (Level III)

23. Holmes GL, Lombroso C. Prognostic value of background patterns in the neonatal EEG. J Clin Neurophysiol 1993;10:323–52. (Level III)

24. Ortibus EL, Sum JM, Hahn JS. Predictive value of EEG for outcome and epilepsy following neonatal seizures. Electroencephalogr Clin Neurophysiol 1996;98:175–85. (Level II-2)

25. Takeuchi T, Watanabe K. The EEG evolution and neurological prognosis of neonates with perinatal hypoxia. Brain Dev 1989;11:115–20. (Level III)

26. Tharp BR, Cukier F, Monod N. The prognostic value of the electroencephalogram in premature infants. Electroencephalogr Clin Neurophysiol 1981;51:219–36. (Level II-2)

27. Sarnat HB, Sarnat MS. Neonatal encephalopathy following fetal distress. A clinical and electroencephalographic study. Arch Neurol 1976;33:696–705. (Level III)

28. Nelson KB, Dambrosia JM, Grether JK, Phillips TM. Neonatal cytokines and coagulation factors in children with cerebral palsy. Ann Neurol 1998;44:666–75. (Level II-2)

29. Nelson KB, Willoughby RE. Infection, inflammation and the risk of cerebral palsy. Curr Opin Neurol 2000;13:133–9. (Level III)

30. Yoon BH, Romero R, Park JS, Kim CJ, Kim SH, Choi JH, et al. Fetal exposure to an intra-amnionic inflammation and the development of cerebral palsy at the age of three years. Am J Obstet Gynecol 2000;182:675–81. (Level II-2)

31. Wu YW, Colford CM Jr. Chorioamnionitis as a risk factor for cerebral palsy. A meta-analysis. JAMA 2000;284:1417–24. (Meta-analysis)

32. Burke CJ, Tannenberg AE. Prenatal brain damage and placental infarction—an autopsy study. Dev Med Child Neurol 1995;37:555–62. (Level III)

33. Grafe MR. The correlation of prenatal brain damage with placental pathology. J Neuropathol Exp Neurol 1994;53:407–15. (Level III)

34. Kraus FT, Acheen VI. Fetal thrombotic vasculopathy in the placenta: cerebral thrombi and infarcts, coagulopathies, and cerebral palsy. Hum Pathol 1999;30:759–69. (Level III)

35. Redline RW, Wilson-Costello D, Borawski E, Fanaroff AA, Hack M. Placental lesions associated with neurologic impairment and cerebral palsy in very low-birth-weight infants. Arch Pathol Lab Med 1998;122:1091–8. (Level II-2)

36. Benirschke K. The contribution of placental anastomoses to prenatal twin damage. Hum Pathol 1992;23:1319–20. (Level III)

37. Hanlon-Lundberg KM, Kirby RS, Gandhi S, Broekhuizen FF. Nucleated red blood cells in cord blood of singleton term neonates. Am J Obstet Gynecol 1997;176:1149–54; discussion 1154–64; discussion 1154–6. (Level II-3)

38. Buonocore G, Perrone S, Gioia D, Gatti MG, Massafra C, Agosta R, et al. Nucleated red blood cell count at birth as an index of perinatal brain damage. Am J Obstet Gynecol 1999;181:1500–5. (Level II-2)

39. Phelan JP, Ahn MO, Korst LM, Martin GI. Nucleated red blood cells: a marker for fetal asphyxia? Am J Obstet Gynecol 1995;173:1380–4. (Level II-2)

40. Korst LM, Phelan JP, Ahn MO, Martin GI. Nucleated red blood cells: an update on the marker for fetal asphyxia. Am J Obstet Gynecol 1996;175:843–6. (Level II-2)

41. Phelan JP, Korst LM, Ahn MO, Martin GI. Neonatal nucleated red blood cell and lymphocyte counts in fetal brain injury. Obstet Gynecol 1998;91:485–9. (Level II-3)

42. Naeye RL, Localio AR. Determining the time before birth when ischemia and hypoxemia initiated cerebral palsy. Obstet Gynecol 1995;86:713–9. (Level II-2)

43. Leikin E, Verma U, Klein S, Tejani N. Relationship between neonatal nucleated red blood cell counts and

hypoxic-ischemic injury. Obstet Gynecol 1996;87: 439–43. (Level II-2)

44. Leikin E, Garry D, Visintainer P, Verma U, Tejani N. Correlation of neonatal nucleated red blood cell counts in preterm infants with histologic chorioamnionitis. Am J Obstet Gynecol 1997;177:27–30. (Level II-2)

45. Ruth V, Autti-Ramo I, Granstrom ML, Korkman M, Raivio KO. Prediction of perinatal brain damage by cord plasma vasopressin, erythropoietin and hypoxanthine values. J Pediatr 1988;113:880–5. (Level II-2)

46. Ruth V, Widness JA, Clemons G, Raivio KO. Postnatal changes in serum immunoreactive erythropoietin in relation to hypoxia before and after birth. J Pediatr 1990;116:950–4. (Level II-2)

47. Maier RF, Bohme K, Dudenhausen JW, Obladen M. Cord blood erythropoietin in relation to different markers of fetal hypoxia. Obstet Gynecol 1993;81: 575–80. (Level II-3)

48. Fonseca E, Garcia-Alonso A, Zarate A, Ochoa R, Galvan RE, Jimenez-Solis G. Elevation of activity of creatine phosphokinase (CK) and its isoenzymes in the newborn is associated with fetal asphyxia and risk at birth. Clin Biochem 1995;28:91–5. (Level II-2)

49. Estan J, Hope P. Unilateral neonatal cerebral infarction in full term infants. Arch Dis Child Fetal Neonatal Ed 1997;76:F88–F93. (Level II-3)

50. deVeber GA, MacGregor D, Curtis R, Mayank S. Neurologic outcome in survivors of childhood arterial ischemic stroke and sinovenous thrombosis. J Child Neurol 2000;15:316–24. (Level II-2)

51. deVeber G, Andrew M, Adams C, Bjornson B, Booth F, Buckley DJ, et al. Cerebral sinovenous thrombosis in children. N Engl J Med 2001;345:417–23. (Level II-2)

52. Uvebrant P. Hemiplegic cerebral palsy. Aetiology and outcome. Acta Paediatr Scand Suppl 1988;345:1–100. (Level III)

53. Humphreys P, Whiting S, Pham B. Hemiparetic cerebral palsy: clinical pattern and imaging in prediction of outcome. Can J Neurol Sci 2000;27:210–9. (Level II-3)

54. Ment LR, Duncan CC, Ehrenkranz RA. Perinatal cerebral infarction. Ann Neurol 1984;16:559–68. (Level III)

55. Yates PO. Birth trauma to the vertebral arteries. Arch Dis Child 1959;34:436–41. (Level III)

56. Clancy R, Malin S, Laraque D, Baumgart S, Younkin D. Focal motor seizures heralding stroke in full-term neonates. Am J Dis Child 1985;139:601–6. (Level III)

57. Filipek PA, Krishnamoorthy KS, Davis KR, Kuehnle K. Focal cerebral infarction in the newborn: a distinct entity. Pediatr Neurol 1987;3:141–7. (Level III)

58. Levy SR, Abroms IF, Marshall PC, Rosquete EE. Seizures and cerebral infarction in the full-term newborn. Ann Neurol 1985;17:366–70. (Level III)

59. Mantovani JF, Gerber GJ. Idiopathic neonatal cerebral infarction. Am J Dis Child 1984;138:359–62. (Level III)

60. Allan WC, Riviello JJ. Perinatal cerebrovascular disease in the neonate. Parenchymal ischemic lesions in term and preterm infants. Pediatr Clin North Am 1992;39:621–50. (Level III)

61. Bouza H, Dubowitz LM, Rutherford M, Pennock JM. Prediction of outcome in children with congenital hemiplegia: a magnetic resonance imaging study. Neuropediatrics 1994;25:60–6. (Level II-3)

62. Golomb MR, MacGregor DL, Domi T, Armstrong DC, McCrindle BW, Mayan KS, et al. Presumed pre- or perinatal arterial ischemic stroke: risk factors and outcomes. Ann Neurol 2001;50:163–8. (Level III)

63. Volpe JJ. Neurology of the newborn. 4th ed. Philadelphia (PA): WB Saunders; 2001. (Level III)

64. Barmada MA, Moossy J, Shuman RM. Cerebral infarcts with arterial occlusion in neonates. Ann of Neurol 1979;6:495–502. (Level II-2)

65. Altshuler G. Some placental considerations related to neurodevelopmental and other disorders. J Child Neurol 1993;8:78–94. (Level III)

66. Amit M, Camfield PR. Neonatal polycythemia causing multiple cerebral infarcts. Arch Neurol 1980;37: 109–10. (Level III)

67. Dominguez R, Aguirre Vila-Coro A, Slopis JM, Bohan TP. Brain and ocular abnormalities in infants with in utero exposure to cocaine and other street drugs. Am J Dis Child 1991;145:688–95. (Level III)

68. Roessmann U, Miller RT. Thrombosis of the middle cerebral artery associated with birth trauma. Neurology 1980;30:889–92. (Level III)

69. Kohlhase B, Vielhaber H, Kehl HG, Kececioglu D, Koch HG, Nowak-Gotti Y. Thromboembolism and resistance to activated protein C in children with underlying cardiac disease. J Pediatr 1996;129:677–9. (Level II-3)

70. Ruff RL, Shaw CM, Beckwith JB, Iozzo RV. Cerebral infarction complicating umbilical vein catheterization. Ann Neurol 1979;6:85. (Level III)

71. Ment LR, Ehrenkranz RA, Duncan CC. Bacterial meningitis as an etiology of perinatal cerebral infarction. Pediatr Neurol 1986;2:276–9. (Level III)

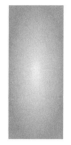

CHAPTER 6

GENETIC, ANATOMIC, AND METABOLIC ETIOLOGIES OF NEONATAL ENCEPHALOPATHY

Dozens of distinct genetic, metabolic, and anatomic factors may contribute to the etiology of neonatal encephalopathy. In many cases, these factors overlap and the distinction between a genetic etiology and a metabolic etiology—both of which can have anatomic consequences—is problematic and pedantic. Furthermore, the timing of onset of signs and symptoms of these disorders varies among and within diagnoses. A systematic discussion of all the possibilities is beyond the scope of this document, but extensive compilations have been published (1–4).

Neonatal abnormalities of brain function, while constituting only a minority of the cases ultimately diagnosed, form an important subset because a number of them are amenable to either palliative or ultimately corrective actions if they are recognized before irreversible damage ensues. The possibility that an infant presenting with classic findings of neonatal encephalopathy may have an etiology secondary to one of these genetic and metabolic causes should prompt an appropriate neonatal investigation before concluding that any problems are related to nongenetic antepartum or peripartum events.

Most of these disorders act by induced abnormalities of metabolism, which result in either hypoglycemia, hyperammonemia, or altered levels of other various brain metabolites. Many of these will then have a detrimental impact on the function and structure of the brain, which can produce irreversible metabolic, physiologic, and anatomic consequences.

Many of the disorders of amino acid metabolism will manifest clinically in the first month of life (Table 6–1). These include the urea-cycle defects, maple syrup urine disease, nonketotic hyperglycinemia, hypervalinemia, methionine malabsorption, phenylketonuria, lysinuric protein intolerance, and pyridoxine dependency. Most of these are autosomal recessive disorders. An example is maple syrup urine disease, which consists of an enzymatic defect involving oxidative decarboxylation of the branched-chain keto acids. Significantly elevated fluid levels of such branched-chain keto acids and branched-chain amino acids yield altered neurotransmitters and impaired energy metabolism (see Box 1). Clinically, this results in vomiting, stupor, seizure, and a specific odor.

Table 6–1. Amino Acid Metabolism Abnormalities Associated with Neurologic Manifestations in the First Month of Life

Disorder	Major Clinical Features	Enzymatic Defect
Urea cycle defects	Vomiting, stupor, and seizures	Carbamyl phosphate synthetase, ornithine transcarbamylase, argininosuccinic acid synthetase, argininosuccinase
Maple syrup urine disease	Stupor, seizures, and odor of maple syrup	Branched-chain keto acid decarboxylase
Nonketotic	Stupor, seizures, and hiccups	Glycine decarboxylase hyperglycinemia
Hypervalinemia	Stupor and delayed development	Valine transaminase
Methionine malabsorption (oasthouse urine disease)	Seizures and odor of hops	Unknown
Phenylketonuria	Vomiting and musty odor	Phenylalanine hydroxylase
Lysinuric protein intolerance	Vomiting and hypotonia	Transport of cationic amino acids (lysine, arginine, ornithine)
Pyridoxine dependency	Seizures	Glutamic acid decarboxylase(pyridoxal phosphate binding site), decreased gamma-aminobutyric acid synthesis

Adapted from Volpe JJ. Hyperammonemia and other disorders of amino acid metabolism. In: Neurology of the newborn. 4th ed. Philadelphia (PA): WB Saunders; 2001. p. 547–73.

Metabolically, it results in acidosis, hypoglycemia, and elevated levels of the branched-chain amino and keto acids. Histologically, it causes myelin and dendritic abnormalities.

In nonketotic hyperglycinemia, the clinical picture includes seizures, stupor, myoclonus, and hiccups. Metabolically, hyperglycinemia occurs, and histologically, myelin disturbance and neuronal excitotoxicity again exist (5, 6) (see Box 2). The major biochemical marker is accumulation of glycine in the blood, urine, and cerebrospinal fluid. Anatomically, the major feature is myelin diminution and vacuolation, thought to be secondary to the hyperglycinemia. Other amino acid abnormalities have been associated with altered neurologic states, including hypervalinemia, methionine malabsorption, phenylketonuria, lysinuric protein intolerance, pyridoxine dependency, hyper-β-alaninemia, sarcosinemia, carnosinemia, and sulfate oxidase deficiency.

Neonatal Hypoglycemia

Studies in animals have shown a correlation between the severity and length of hypoglycemia and the degree of neuronal damage. Human data suggest this correlation may apply to humans as well (7, 8). Hypoglycemia results in neuronal injury, as well as injury to the glia. Severe recurrent hypoglycemia is caused by several metabolic and endocrine abnormalities involving glucose control. A number of conditions produce hyperinsulinism, endocrine deficiencies, or hereditary metabolic defects (9–13) that have a primary result of persistent neonatal hypoglycemia (see Box 3).

Hyperammonemia

There are multiple disorders of amino acid metabolism (14) whose primary result is the major accumulation of ammonia. The clinical picture from hyperammonemia includes seizures, hypotonia, vomiting, altered level of consciousness, and delayed neurologic development.

The most common causes of hyperammonemia are the urea cycle defects, including carbamyl phosphatase, ornithine transcarbamylase, argininosuccinic acid synthetase, and argininosuccinase deficiencies (15) (see Box 4). These disorders principally alter hepatic enzyme function and secondarily affect certain other enzymes. However, the principal defect is an increased level of ammonia, which impairs conversion of pyruvate to citrate. With declining brain aspartate levels, potentiation of gamma-aminobutyric acid responses increases brain glutamine synthesis, which in turn increases tryptophan transport into the brain and metabolism to serotonin and quinolinic acid. Astrocytic swelling is induced, which impairs glutamate uptake and leads to microcirculatory disturbances and glutamate excitatory injury (see Box 5).

Other disorders can likewise produce hyperammonemia, including propionic acidemia, methylmalonic aciduria, β-ketothiolase deficiency, isovaleric acidemia, glutaric aciduria, multiple carboxylase deficiency, pyruvate dehydrogenate deficiency, and fatty-acid oxidation defects.

Organic Acid Abnormalities

Organic acid abnormalities are significant causes of severe, neonatal metabolic acidosis (15). Many genetic etiologies have relevant neurologic components with deleterious effects on the developing central nervous system (see Box 6). Common features include vomiting, tachypnea, stupor, and seizures, with a profound metabolic acidosis and pathologically produced myelin disturbances. Brain injury comes from lactic acidosis.

Degenerative Diseases

A number of degenerative disorders of the developing central nervous system can have clinical manifestations, even in the neonatal period (16, 17). Most are related to metabolic abnormalities of lipids or other compounds and are autosomal recessive disorders. For some, therapy is possible. Many of these, such as Tay–Sachs disease, classically do not present in the newborn period but, periodically, manifestations may be seen. Multiple examples have been categorized principally by those affecting gray matter, white matter, and combinations of both (see Box 7). Many of these disorders have characteristic neuropathologic findings that commonly explain the clinical manifestations seen.

Lower Motor Neurons

Lower motor neuron disorders are causes of severe hypotonia and weakness in the neonatal

---

Box 1. Branched-Chain Amino Acid and Keto Acid Disorders and Their Sequelae

Impaired energy metabolism
- Hypoglycemia
- Decreased pyruvate decarboxylation to acetylcoenzyme A
- Increased lactate
- Decreased cerebral oxygen consumption

Impaired protein synthesis
- Disturbed transport of amino acids
- Decreased aminoacyl-soluble ribonucleic acid (sRNA) synthesis

Impaired myelin formation
- Decreased myelin lipid synthesis
- Decreased proteolipid protein synthesis

Alteration of neurotransmitters
- Decreased gamma-aminobutyric acid
- Decreased serotonin

Adapted from Volpe JJ. Hyperammonemia and other disorders of amino acid metabolism. In: Neurology of the newborn. 4th ed. Philadelphia (PA): WB Saunders; 2001. p. 547–73.

Box 2. Nonketotic Hyperglycinemia (Glycine Encephalopathy)

Clinical features
- Seizures
- Stupor, coma
- Myoclonus
- Hiccups

Metabolic results
- Hyperglycinemia (hyperglycinuria)

Neuropathologic consequences
- Myelin disturbance
- Neuronal excitotoxicity

Adapted from Volpe JJ. Hyperammonemia and other disorders of amino acid metabolism. In: Neurology of the newborn. 4th ed. Philadelphia (PA): WB Saunders; 2001. p. 547–73.

period (18). Werdnig-Hoffman disease is the most common, although the differential diagnosis of lower motor neuron hypotonia and weakness includes neurogenic arthrogryposis, glycogen storage disease type II, hypoxic–ischemic injury, and neonatal poliomyelitis (see Box 8). Likewise, a number of neuronal migration disorders present like cerebral palsy (see Box 9).

Box 3. Examples of Severe, Recurrent, or Persistent Neonatal Hypoglycemia Conditions

Endocrine deficiencies
- Panhypopituitarism
- Isolated growth hormone deficiency
- Cortisol deficiency (adrenocorticotropic hormone unresponsiveness, isolated glucocorticoid deficiency, maternal steroid therapy, adrenal hemorrhage, adrenogenital syndrome)
- Hypothyroidism
- Glucagon deficiency

Hyperinsulinism
- Beckwith-Wiedemann syndrome
- Macrosomia (without Beckwith-Weidemann syndrome)
- β-cell nesidioblastosis—adenoma spectrum
- Functional β-cell hyperplasia (without nesidioblastosis or adenoma)
- Leucine sensitivity

Hereditary metabolic defects
- Carbohydrate metabolism (galactosemia, glucose-6-phosphatase deficiency [von Gierke disease], glycogen synthetase deficiency, fructose-1,6-diphosphatase deficiency, phosphoenolpyruvate carboxykinase deficiency, pyruvate carboxylase deficiency)
- Amino acid metabolism (maple syrup urine disease, hereditary tyrosinemia)
- Organic acid metabolism (propionic acidemia, methylmalonic acidemia)
- Fatty-acid metabolism (medium- and long-chain acyl-CoA dehydrogenase deficiencies)

Adapted from Volpe JJ. Hypoglycemia and brain injury. In: Neurology of the newborn. 4th ed. Philadelphia (PA): WB Saunders; 2001. p. 497–520.

Primary Anatomic Abnormalities

Most anatomic abnormalities, either at the macroscopic or microscopic level, involved in neonatal encephalopathy are related to metabolic alterations (19). However, profound anatomic disturbances, such as porencephalic cysts, encephaloceles, hydrocephalus (with or without associated myelomeningocele), and hydranencephaly, all produce abnormalities of neurologic circuitry and functioning. Many of these, such as the neural tube defects, are multifactorial and polygenic in origin.

Chromosome Abnormalities

Several chromosome abnormalities, such as trisomy 13, trisomy 18, and triploidy, show imme-

---

Box 4. Etiologies of Hyperammonemia in the Neonatal Period

Organic acid disorders
- Propionic acidemia
- Methylmalonic acidemia
- Isovaleric acidemia
- β-ketothiolase deficiency
- Pyruvate dehydrogenase deficiency
- Mitochondrial (electron transport) disorders
- Glutaric aciduria, type II
- Multiple carboxylase deficiency
- Fatty-acid oxidation defect

Urea cycle defects
- Carbamyl phosphate synthetase
- Ornithine transcarbamylase
- Argininosuccinic acid synthetase
- Argininosuccinase

Lysine protein intolerance

Hyperornithinemia, hyperammonemia, and homocitrullinemia

Transient hyperammonemia of prematurity

Perinatal asphyxia

Adapted from Volpe JJ. Hyperammonemia and other disorders of amino acid metabolism. In: Neurology of the newborn. 4th ed. Philadelphia (PA): WB Saunders; 2001. p. 547–73.

diate profound neurologic sequelae in the newborn period. Others, such as trisomy 21, show more subtle functional abnormalities.

Altered Susceptibility to External Forces

It has long been appreciated that there are different degrees of genetic resistance and susceptibility to external forces. In many cases, these may be clinically unrecognizable. However, population-based studies demonstrate that the incidence of neural tube defects (and resulting neurologic sequelae) is in fact ethnically derived (20, 21).

Box 5. Pathophysiology of Neurologic Dysfunction and Injury with Congenital Hyperammonemia

Toxic effects of ammonia
- Impaired conversion of pyruvate to citrate, with decrease in brain aspartate level
- Potentiation of gamma-aminobutyric acid responses
- Increase in brain glutamine synthesis from glutamate
- Deleterious effects of glutamine:
  —Increased tryptophan transport into brain and metabolism to serotonin and quinolinic acid (excitotoxin at N-methyl-D-aspartate receptor)
  —Induction of astrocytic swelling and thereby impairment of glutamate uptake, microcirculatory disturbance, and glutamate-excitotoxic injury
- Impaired transport of reducing equivalents (reduced nicotinamide adenine dinucleotide) from cytosol to mitochondrion (late)
- Impaired energy production (late)
- Accumulation of amino acid(s) proximal to an enzymatic block or related metabolites or both, which may be toxic
- Deficiency of amino acid(s) distal to an enzymatic block or of related metabolites or both, which may be necessary for normal central nervous system structure and function

Adapted from Volpe JJ. Hyperammonemia and other disorders of amino acid metabolism. In: Neurology of the newborn. 4th ed. Philadelphia (PA): WB Saunders; 2001. p. 547–73.

Box 6. Etiologies of Metabolic Acidosis in the Neonatal Period

Disorders of pyruvate metabolism and mitochondrial energy metabolism
- Pyruvate dehydrogenase deficiency
- Pyruvate carboxylase deficiency
- Defects of the electron transport chain (complexes I, III, IV, V)

Disorders of propionate-methylmalonate metabolism
- Propionic acidemia
- Methylmalonic acidemia

Disorders of branched-chain amino acid-keto acid metabolism
- Maple syrup urine disease
- Isovaleric acidemia
- β-Methylcrotonyl-coenzyme A carboxylase deficiency
- β-Ketothiolase deficiency
- 3-Hydroxy-3-methylglutaryl coenzyme A lyase deficiency
- Mevalonic aciduria

Disorders of fatty-acid metabolism
- Medium-chain acyl-coenzyme A dehydrogenase deficiency

Other organic acid disorders
- Multiple carboxylase deficiency
- Glutaric acidemia, type II
- Glutathione synthetase deficiency (5-oxoprolinuria)
- Sulfite oxidase deficiency (molybdenum cofactor deficiency)

Disorders of carbohydrate metabolism
- Galactosemia
- Glycogen storage disease, type I (von Gierke glucose-6-phosphatase deficiency)
- Fructose-1,6-diphosphatase deficiency
- Phosphoenolpyruvate carboxykinase deficiency

Renal tubular acidosis

Adapted from Volpe JJ. Disorders of organic acid metabolism. In: Neurology of the newborn. 4th ed. Philadelphia (PA): WB Saunders; 2001. p. 574–98.

Box 7. Degenerative Diseases of the Nervous System with Manifestations in the Newborn

White matter
- Canavan disease
- Alexander's disease
- Krabbe's disease
- Pelizaeus-Merzbacher disease
- Metachromatic leukodystrophy
- Leukodystrophy with cerebral calcifications

Gray matter
- No visceral storage
  —Tay–Sachs disease (GM$_2$ gangliosidosis)
  —Congenital or early infantile neuronal ceroid-lipofuscinosis
  —Alpers' disease
  —Menkes' syndrome
- With visceral storage
  —GM$_1$ gangliosidosis
  —GM$_2$ gangliosidosis (Sandhoff variant)
  —Niemann-Pick disease
  —Gaucher's disease
  —Farber's disease
  —Infantile sialic acid storage disease

Gray and White Matter
- Peroxisomal disorders—Neonatal adrenoleukodystrophy or Zellweger syndrome
- Mitochondrial disorder—Leigh disease
- Cytoskeletal disorder—Infantile neuroaxonal dystrophy

Adapted from Volpe JJ. Degenerative diseases of the newborn. In: Neurology of the newborn. 4th ed. Philadelphia (PA): WB Saunders; 2001. p. 599–619.

Box 8. Hypotonia and Weakness— Level of the Lower Motor Neuron

Werdnig-Hoffmann disease

Neurogenic arthrogryposis multiplex congenita

Glycogen storage disease, type II (Pompe's disease)

Hypoxic–ischemic injury

Neonatal poliomyelitis (other enteroviruses)

Adapted from Volpe JJ. Neuromuscular disorders: levels above the lower motor neuron to the neuromuscular junction. In: Neurology of the newborn. 4th ed. Philadelphia (PA): WB Saunders; 2001. p. 642–70.

The highest incidence in the world is in Northern Ireland (22) and Northern China (23), while the incidence among African and Asian patients is substantially lower (24, 25). Folic acid may exert a beneficial external influence on this incidence, particularly in patients with a variant of methylenetetrahydrofolate reductase (21). Such differences may exist for the neurologic sequelae of these disorders and also in the resistance to insult from other genetically derived and externally

Box 9. Syndromes Associated with Neuronal Migration Disorders that May Be Described as Cerebral Palsy

Metabolic
- Zellweger syndrome
- Glutaric aciduria, type II
- Gangliosidosis

Chromosomal
- Trisomies 13, 18
- Deletion 4p, 17p13 (Miller-Dieker syndrome)

Neuromuscular
- Walker-Warburg syndrome
- Myotonic dystrophy

Neurocutaneous
- Neurofibromatosis type I
- Encephalocranial cutaneous lipomatosis
- Tuberous sclerosis
- Epidermal nevus syndrome

Multiple Congenital Anomalies
- Smith-Lemli-Opitz syndrome
- Potter's syndrome
- Cornelia de Lange's syndrome
- Oculo-renal-cerebellar syndrome

Other Central Nervous System Dysplasias
- Aicardi's syndrome
- Joubert's syndrome
- Hemimegalencephaly
- Atelencephaly
- Congenital rubella syndrome
- Fetal cytomegalovirus infection
- Fetal iodine deficiency
- Fetal methylmercury poisoning

Adapted from Stanley F, Blair E, Alberman E. Causal pathways initiated preconceptually or early in pregnancy. In: Cerebral palsies: epidemiology and causal pathways. New London: Mac Keith Press; 2000. p. 48–59.

derived abnormalities seen with the numerous genetic diseases listed in this chapter. It is unlikely that a realistic way of quantifying these differences will emerge in the near future, but with better understanding of the pathophysiology, including genetic susceptibility, it may be possible to understand why certain fetuses are more susceptible to toxic agents than others.

Looking to the future, with the emergence of molecular technologies and knowledge derived from the human genome, we may come to an understanding of how external forces, such as infection, interact with the genetic composition of individual fetuses. Thus, it is highly likely we will learn why the same insult is irrelevant to some and devastating to others.

Conclusions

- A family history should be part of any evaluation for neonatal encephalopathy.

- There are a large number of genetic, metabolic, and anatomic factors that can contribute to the etiology of neonatal encephalopathy. However, such causes clearly constitute only a small proportion of all cases. Although these causes should ideally be considered, such investigation will be fruitful only in a small percentage of cases.

References

1. Badawi N, Watson L, Petterson B, Blair E, Slee J, Haan E, et al. What constitutes cerebral palsy? Dev Med Child Neurol 1998;40:520–7. (Level III)

2. Burton BK. Inborn errors of metabolism in infancy: a guide to diagnosis. Pediatrics 1998;102:E69. (Level III)

3. Volpe JJ. Neurology of the newborn. 4th ed. Philadelphia (PA): WB Saunders; 2001. (Level III)

4. Stanley F, Blair E, Alberman E. Causal pathways initiated preconceptionally or in early pregnancy. In: Cerebral palsies: epidemiology and causal pathways. London: Mac Keith Press; 2000. p. 48–59. (Level III)

5. Langan TJ, Pueschel SM. Nonketotic hyperglycemia: clinical, biochemical and therapeutic considerations. Curr Probl Pediatr 1983;13:1–30. (Level III)

6. Hamosh A, Johnston MV. Nonketotic hyperglycinemia. In: Scriver CR, Beaudet AL, Sly WS, Valle D, editors. The metabolic and molecular bases of inherited disease. Vol 2. 8th ed. New York: McGraw-Hill; 2001. p. 2065–78. (Level III)

7. Anderson JM, Milner RD, Strich SJ. Effects of neonatal hypoglycaemia on the nervous system: a pathological study. J Neurol Neurosurg Psychiatry 1967;30: 295–310. (Level III)

8. Griffiths AD, Laurence KM. The effect of hypoxia and hypoglycaemia on the brain of the newborn human infant. Dev Med Child Neurol 1974;16:308–19. (Level II-3)

9. Menni F, de Lonlay P, Sevin C, Touati G, Peigne C, Barbier V, et al. Neurologic outcomes of 90 neonates and infants with persistent hyperinsulinemic hypoglycemia. Pediatrics 2001;107:476–9. (Level II-3)

10. De Lonlay P, Benelli C, Fouque F, Ganguly A, Aral B, Dionisi-Vici C, et al. Hyperinsulinism and hyperammonemia syndrome: report of twelve unrelated patients. Pediatr Res 2001;50:353–7. (Level III)

11. Kauschansky A, Genel M, Smith GJ. Congenital hypopituitarism in female infants. Its association with hypoglycemia and hypothyroidism. Am J Dis Child 1979;133:165–9. (Level III)

12. Vockley J, Whiteman DA. Defects of mitochondrial beta-oxidation: a growing group of disorders. Neuromuscul Discord 2002;12:235–46. (Level III)

13. Ozand PT. Hypoglycemia in association with various organic and amino acid disorders. Semin Perinatol 2000;24:172–93. (Level III)

14. Summar M, Tuchman M. Proceedings of a consensus conference for the management of patients with urea cycle disorders. J Pediatr 2001;138:S6–10. (Level III)

15. Mahoney MJ. Organic acidemias. Clin Perinatol 1976;3:61–78. (Level III)

16. Powers JM, Rubio A. Selected leukodystrophies. Semin Pediatr Neurol 1995;2:200–10. (Level III)

17. Vadasz AG, Epstein LG. Degenerative central nervous system disease. Pediatr Rev 1995;16:426–31. (Level III)

18. Rudnik-Schoneborn S, Forkert R, Hahnen E, Wirth B, Zerres K. Clinical spectrum and diagnostic criteria of infantile spinal muscular atrophy: further delineation on the basis of SMN gene deletion findings. Neuropediatrics 1996;27:8–15. (Level III)

19. Felix JF, Badawi N, Kurinczuk JJ, Bower C, Keogh JM, Pemberton PJ. Birth defects in children with newborn encephalopathy. Dev Med Child Neurol 2000; 42:803–8. (Level II-2)

20. Mutchinick OM, Lopez MA, Luna L, Waxman J, Babinsky VE. High prevalence of the thermolabile methylenetetrahydrofolate reductase variant in Mexico: a country with a very high prevalence of neural tube defects. Mol Genet Metab 1999;68:461–7. (Level II-3)

21. Shields DC, Kirke PN, Mills JL, Ramsbottom D, Molloy AM, Burke H, et al. The "thermolabile" variant of methylenetetrahydrofolate reductase and neural tube defects: an evaluation of genetic risk and the relative importance of the genotypes of the embryo and

the mother. Am J Hum Genet 1999;64:1045–55. (Level II-2)

22. Nevin NC, Johnston WP. A family study of spina bifida and anencephalus in Belfast, Northern Ireland (1964 to 1968). J Med Genet 1980;17:203–11. (Level III)

23. Moore CA, Li S, Li Z, Hong SX, Gu HQ, Berry RJ, et al. Elevated rates of severe neural tube defects in a high-prevalence area in northern China. Am J Med Genet 1997;73:113–8. (Level II-2)

24. Berry RJ, Li Z, Erickson JD, Li S, Moore CA, Wang H, et al. Prevention of neural-tube defects with folic acid in China. China-U.S. Collaborative Project for Neural Tube Defect Prevention. N Engl J Med 1999; 341:1485–90. (Level II-2)

25. Ehara H, Ohno K, Ohtani K, Koeda T, Takeshita K. Epidemiology of spina bifida in Tottori Prefecture, Japan, 1976–1995. Pediatr Neurol 1998;19:199–203. (Level III)

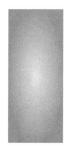

CHAPTER 7

OBSTETRIC PHARMACOLOGIC APPROACHES TO THE PREVENTION OF NEONATAL HYPOXIC–ISCHEMIC ENCEPHALOPATHY: CURRENT STATUS AND FUTURE DIRECTIONS

Current Status

At present, there are no data to support that neonatal encephalopathy or its subtype hypoxic–ischemic encephalopathy can be prevented or the consequences mitigated by maternal administration of a pharmacologic agent. Specifically, no observational studies report an association between maternal receipt of a pharmacologic agent(s) and a decreased risk or improved outcome of neonatal encephalopathy. As a result, no clinical trials have been conducted to test the hypothesis that maternal pharmacotherapy might benefit fetuses at risk of neonatal encephalopathy. Although several drugs are promising candidates for treating neonatal encephalopathy, to date only neonates, not fetuses, have been targeted for therapy (1).

Future Directions

Precedents for an Obstetric Pharmacologic Approach

Maternal drug administration for the purpose of fetal neuroprotection does have precedent, both on a research and a clinical level. For instance, maternal phenobarbital as a means of preventing intraventricular hemorrhage in preterm infants has been evaluated in clinical trials but was found to be ineffective (2). On the other hand, clinical trials have found that the glucocorticoids betamethasone and dexamethasone, administered to mothers at risk for preterm birth, protect against neonatal intraventricular hemorrhage (3). Antenatal exposure to betamethasone (but not dexamethasone) has been associated with a decreased risk of cystic periventricular leukomalacia among very preterm infants (4). Finally, observational studies (5, 6) have reported a markedly reduced risk of cerebral palsy in children who were born preterm to women who had received magnesium sulfate before delivery (2). This intriguing association has biologic plausibility and has led to an ongoing study by the National Institutes of Health (the Beneficial Aspects of Antenatal Magnesium or BEAM Trial). A similar trial is underway in Australia. The efficacy of maternally administered magnesium sulfate to decrease either short- or long-term morbidity to the fetus or neonate is yet to be established, and magnesium sulfate's utilization for this purpose remains investigational.

Feasibility of an Obstetric Preventive Approach

If a promising pharmacologic agent for the prevention of neonatal encephalopathy were available and could be administered to the mother, there are factors suggesting that evaluation in a randomized, controlled clinical trial would be extremely difficult. The prevalence of neonatal encephalopathy, while not known precisely, is low. Collectively, neonatal encephalopathy of any etiology has been estimated to occur at a rate of 2–8 births per 1,000 term infants in the first day of life (7). However, evidence of significant intrapartum hypoxia is lacking in more than 70% of cases of neonatal encephalopathy (8). Therefore, neonatal encephalopathy in the term or near-term neonate that is the result of only intrapartum asphyxia likely occurs at a rate of only 1.6 per 10,000 infants in developed countries (8). Studying unselected term pregnancies would require exposing approximately 999 mothers and fetuses to an investigational drug for the benefit of, at most, one fetus. Safety would be an overwhelming concern and such a study would prove to be both scientifically and ethically problematic.

Conclusion

- At this time, and in the foreseeable future, there are no useful pharmacologic measures to prevent or improve the outcome of neonatal encephalopathy.

References

1. Robertson NJ, Edwards AD. Recent advances in developing neuroprotective strategies for perinatal asphyxia. Curr Opin Pediatr 1998;10:575–80. (Level III)

2. Shankaran S, Papile LA, Wright LL, Ehrenkranz RA, Mele L, Lemons JA, et al. The effect of antenatal phenobarbital therapy on neonatal intracranial hemorrhage in preterm infants. N Engl J Med 1997;337: 466–71. (Level I)

3. Crowley P. Prophylactic corticosteroids for preterm birth. (Cochrane Review.) In: The Cochrane Library, Issue 4, 2001. Oxford: Update Software. (Meta-analysis)

4. Baud O, Foix-L'Helias L, Kaminski M, Audibert F, Jarreau P, Papiernik E, et al. Antenatal glucocorticoid treatment and cystic periventricular leukomalacia in very premature infants. N Engl J Med 1999;341: 1190–6. (Level II-2)

5. Nelson KB, Grether JK. Can magnesium sulfate reduce the risk of cerebral palsy in very low birth-weight infants? Pediatrics 1995;95:263–9. (Level II-2)

6. Schendel DE, Berg CJ, Yeargin-Allsopp M, Boyle CA, Decoufle P. Prenatal magnesium sulfate exposure and the risk for cerebral palsy or mental retardation among very low-birth-weight children aged 3 to 5 years. JAMA 1996;276:1805–10. (Level II-2)

7. Leviton A, Nelson KB. Problems with definitions and classifications of newborn encephalopathy. Pediatr Neurol 1992;8:85–90. (Level III)

8. Badawi N, Kurinczuk JJ, Keogh JM, Alessandri LM, O'Sullivan F, Burton PR, et al. Intrapartum risk factors for newborn encephalopathy: the Western Australian case-control study. BMJ 1998;317:1554–8. (Level II-2)

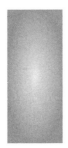

CHAPTER 8

CRITERIA REQUIRED TO DEFINE AN ACUTE INTRAPARTUM HYPOXIC EVENT AS SUFFICIENT TO CAUSE CEREBRAL PALSY

Careful analysis of data compiled over the past 25 years demonstrates that intrapartum complications are less common causes of cerebral palsy than previously thought. Clinical epidemiologic studies indicate that in most cases the events leading to cerebral palsy occur as a result of multifactorial and unpreventable reasons either during fetal development or in the newborn after delivery (1–8).

See box for a description of the criteria required to define an acute intrapartum hypoxic event as sufficient to cause cerebral palsy. This box is a modification and update of the International Cerebral Palsy Task Force Consensus Statement, *A template for defining a causal relation between acute intrapartum events and cerebral palsy*, published in the British Medical Journal in 1999 (9).

Part 1.1 of the criteria presents four essential criteria that are necessary before an intrapartum hypoxic event can be considered as a cause of cerebral palsy. If any 1 of the 4 essential criteria is not met, this provides strong evidence that intrapartum hypoxia was not the cause of cerebral palsy. When all four essential criteria outlined are met, it is then important to determine whether the hypoxia is attributable to chronic or intermittent hypoxia of long standing duration of days or weeks or whether acute hypoxia has occurred during labor in a previously healthy fetus.

Part 1.2 of the criteria presents a set of five criteria that collectively suggest an intrapartum timing. With the exception of the first criteria of an acute hypoxic sentinel event occurring immediately before or during labor, all four other criteria described are weakly associated with acute intrapartum hypoxia. It is not necessary for all five of these criteria to be present to establish the relationship between acute intrapartum hypoxia and cerebral palsy. Accordingly, contrary evidence such as a reassuring fetal heart pattern, a normal Apgar score of 7 or greater at 5 minutes, or an early magnetic resonance imaging (MRI) study inconsistent with a recent global hypoxic or ischemic event excludes an injurious event during labor.

The use of these criteria will help to evaluate the probability that the pathology causing the cerebral palsy occurred during labor. For additional information on these criteria, see preceding sections in Chapters 1–7.

Criteria to Define an Acute Intrapartum Hypoxic Event as Sufficient to Cause Cerebral Palsy

1.1: Essential criteria (must meet all four)

1. Evidence of a metabolic acidosis in fetal umbilical cord arterial blood obtained at delivery (pH <7 and base deficit ≥12 mmol/L)

2. Early onset of severe or moderate neonatal encephalopathy in infants born at 34 or more weeks of gestation

3. Cerebral palsy of the spastic quadriplegic or dyskinetic type*

4. Exclusion of other identifiable etiologies, such as trauma, coagulation disorders, infectious conditions, or genetic disorders

1.2: Criteria that collectively suggest an intrapartum timing (within close proximity to labor and delivery, eg, 0–48 hours) but are nonspecific to asphyxial insults

1. A sentinel (signal) hypoxic event occurring immediately before or during labor

2. A sudden and sustained fetal bradycardia or the absence of fetal heart rate variability in the presence of persistent, late, or variable decelerations, usually after a hypoxic sentinel event when the pattern was previously normal

3. Apgar scores of 0–3 beyond 5 minutes

4. Onset of multisystem involvement within 72 hours of birth

5. Early imaging study showing evidence of acute nonfocal cerebral abnormality

*Spastic quadriplegia and, less commonly, dyskinetic cerebral palsy are the only types of cerebral palsy associated with acute hypoxic intrapartum events. Spastic quadriplegia is not specific to intrapartum hypoxia. Hemiparetic cerebral palsy, hemiplegic cerebral palsy, spastic diplegia, and ataxia are unlikely to result from acute intrapartum hypoxia (Nelson KB, Grether JK. Potentially asphyxiating conditions and spastic cerebral palsy in infants of normal birth weight. Am J Obstet Gynecol 1998;179:507–13.).

Modified from MacLennan A. A template for defining a causal relation between acute intrapartum events and cerebral palsy: international consensus statement. BMJ 1999;319:1054–9.

Part 1.1: Essential criteria (must meet all four)

1. Evidence of a metabolic acidosis in fetal umbilical cord arterial blood obtained at delivery (pH <7 and base deficit of ≥12 mmol/L)

It has been demonstrated that a realistic pH threshold for significant pathologic fetal acidemia (ie, a pH associated with adverse neonatal sequelae) is less than 7 (10–13). The metabolic component (ie, base deficit and bicarbonate) is the most important variable associated with subsequent neonatal morbidity in newborns with an umbilical artery pH of less than 7 (14). A base deficit of 12 mmol/L or greater is a reasonable cutoff criterion (15). Metabolic acidemia at birth must be present to establish that a potentially damaging intrapartum hypoxic event is a cause of cerebral palsy. The presence of metabolic acidemia does not define the timing of the onset of the hypoxic event. It is important to remember that even when this pH threshold of less than 7 is used to define significant acidemia, most newborns in this category will be neurologically normal with no apparent morbidity (16, 17).

2. Early onset of severe or moderate neonatal encephalopathy in infants born at 34 or more weeks of gestation

Neonatal encephalopathy is a clinically defined syndrome of disturbed neurologic function in the earliest days of life in the near-term and term infant. If an intrapartum insult is severe enough to result in ischemic cerebral injury, abnormalities will be noted in the neurologic examination within 24 hours after birth. The examination is characterized by abnormalities in 1) cortical function (lethargy, stupor, coma with or without seizures), 2) brainstem function (ie, pupillary and cranial nerve abnormalities), 3) tone (hypotonia), and 4) reflexes (absent, hyporeflexia) (18, 19). Outcome is related to the maximum grade of severity (18). Thus, for infants with mild encephalopathy (stage 1), outcome is invariably favorable; moderate encephalopathy (stage 2) is associated with an abnormal outcome in approximately 20–25% of cases; severe encephalopathy (stage 3) is associated with a poor outcome in all cases (19).

Many cases of severe neonatal encephalopathy are not associated with intrapartum hypoxia (3, 4, 7, 20). The incidence of neonatal encephalopathy attributed to intrapartum hypoxia, in the absence of any other preconceptional or antepartum abnormalities, is estimated to be approximately 1.6 per 10,000 infants.

3. Cerebral palsy of the spastic quadriplegic or dyskinetic type

Spastic quadriplegia and, less commonly, dyskinetic cerebral palsy are the only types of cerebral palsy associated with acute hypoxic intrapartum events (21, 22). Although spastic quadriplegia is the most common subtype of cerebral palsy associated with acute hypoxic intrapartum events, it is not specific to intrapartum hypoxia (22). Unilateral brain lesions are not the result of birth asphyxia; studies relating birth complications to neurologic outcome indicate that hemiparetic cerebral palsy is not a result of known intrapartum asphyxial complications (23, 24). Neither hemiplegic cerebral palsy, spastic diplegia, nor ataxia have been associated with acute intrapartum hypoxia (24). Any progressive neurologic disability is by definition not cerebral palsy and is not associated with acute hypoxic intrapartum events.

There is increasing information concerning another set of risk factors predisposing to fetal and neonatal strokes and thereby to hemiparetic cerebral palsy or, if bilateral, to spastic quadriparetic cerebral palsy (25–27). Such perinatal strokes commonly involve the middle cerebral artery, and many are related to inherited thrombophilias (of which the most common is the factor V Leiden mutation) (28), acquired disorders including antiphospholipid antibodies (29), combinations of these, or with environmental triggers (30).

Thromboembolic disease of the mother can be associated with obstetric complications and may be accompanied by placental thrombosis (31). Embolization from the placenta into the fetal circulation is a probable intermediary event (32).

4. Exclusion of other identifiable etiologies, such as trauma, coagulation disorders, infectious conditions, or genetic disorders

A large proportion of cerebral palsy cases are associated with maternal and antenatal factors, such as preterm birth, intrauterine growth restriction, intrauterine infection, maternal or fetal coagulation disorders, multiple pregnancy, antepartum hemorrhage, breech presentation, and chromosomal or congenital abnormalities (1, 2, 6, 24, 33). These causes must be considered and excluded before concluding intrapartum hypoxia is the cause of cerebral palsy.

Infections and inflammations along with thromboses and coagulopathies are recognized as being associated with white-matter damage and cerebral palsy. Correlates of fetal infection include elevated fetal cytokines in both amniotic fluid and fetal blood. Research in animals and humans has shown an association between inflammatory markers and periventricular leukomalacia and neonatal encephalopathy (34–38).

Coagulation disorders such as antithrombin-III deficiency, abnormalities of protein C or protein S, prothrombin genetic deficiencies, and the factor V Leiden mutation, can lead to stroke (31, 39–41). Also, occlusion of either arterial supply or venous return can cause permanent focal damage. Such damage may rarely be secondary to trauma in pregnancy, especially if in conjunction with an existing coagulation disorder. Early imaging studies may be very useful in identifying and evaluating a specific etiology (42–48).

Numerous genetic and metabolic disorders can present clinically as neonatal encephalopathy; however, although there are many possible genetic causes, in most infants with neonatal encephalopathy, the condition does not result from an identifiable genetic cause, and diagnosis in the perinatal period is unlikely unless there is heightened clinical suspicion based on specific findings or family history. The practitioner should attempt to identify such disorders by taking a family history, performing a thorough examination of the infant for dysmorphic features consistent with a genetic etiology, and ordering appropriate laboratory studies if warranted.

Part 1.2: Criteria that collectively suggest an intrapartum timing (within close proximity to labor and delivery, eg, 0–48 hours) but are nonspecific to asphyxial insults

1. A sentinel (signal) hypoxic event occurring immediately before or during labor

A serious pathologic event has to occur for a neurologically intact fetus to sustain a neurologically damaging acute insult. Examples of such sentinel events include a ruptured uterus, placental abruption, umbilical cord prolapse, amniotic fluid embolus, maternal cardiopulmonary arrest, and fetal exsanguination from either vasoprevia or massive fetomaternal hemorrhage. Any of these events may result in neurologic morbidity and mortality. The result of each insult, however, is not certain and depends on a variety of poorly understood factors. Normal outcomes have been reported following prolonged hypoxia; therefore, a dose response association between the magnitude of hypoxia and neurologic damage is not always present.

2. A sudden and sustained fetal bradycardia or the absence of fetal heart rate variability in the presence of persistent, late, or variable decelerations, usually after an hypoxic sentinel event when the pattern was previously normal

The Task Force endorses the statement by the National Institute of Child Health and Human Development's Research Planning Workshop on electronic fetal heart rate monitoring (49) which presented recommendations for standardized definitions of fetal heart rate tracings. With two exceptions, Workshop members had difficulty reaching consensus on appropriate definitions of certain heart rate patterns. The first exception is the definition of a normal fetal heart pattern as a baseline heart rate within the normal range (110–160 beats per minute) and normal fetal heart rate variability (6–25 beats per minute), presence of accelerations and absence of decelerations. Such a tracing confers an extremely high predictability of a normally oxygenated fetus. The second exception is the agreement among most Workshop members that a fetus with absent fetal heart rate variability in the presence of recurrent late or variable decelerations or a substantial bradycardia has evidence of current or impending damaging acidemia. The Task Force further decided that, because of insufficient evidence, it is impossible to reach consensus on the presumed fetal condition and obstetric management of all other patterns intermediate between the two described previously. Recommendations will have to await further research on the reliability, validity, and ability of monitoring as a means of avoiding adverse outcomes by prompting obstetric action.

The most frequently observed fetal heart rate patterns associated with cerebral palsy are those with multiple late decelerations and decreased beat-to-beat variability. However, these patterns cannot be used to predict cerebral palsy as they have a false positive rate of 99% (50). The high frequency (up to 79%) of nonreassuring patterns found during electronic monitoring of normal pregnancies in labor with normal fetal outcomes make both the decision on the optimal management of the labor and the prediction of current or future neurologic status very difficult (51).

3. Apgar scores of 0–3 beyond 5 minutes

The Apgar score is a quick method of assessing the clinical status of the newborn (52, 53). It is well established that the 1- or 5-minute Apgar score is a poor predictor of long-term neurologic outcome in the individual patient (54). For example, three fourths of children with cerebral palsy have normal Apgar scores (54).

There is good correlation between an extremely low Apgar score at 15 and 20 minutes and subsequent neurologic dysfunction. A score of less than 3 at 15 minutes was associated with a 53% mortality rate and a 36% cerebral palsy rate. When a low score persisted at 20 minutes, mortality was almost 60% and more than one half (57%) of survivors had cerebral palsy (54). The correlation between low Apgar score (<3) and neurologic disability improves somewhat at 10, 15, and 20 minutes after birth. For example, 17% of newborns with 10-minute scores of less than 3 had cerebral palsy, but even in this group, the rate decreased to approximately 5% if the score improved at 15 and 20 minutes (54).

4. Onset of multisystem involvement within 72 hours of birth

Acute hypoxia sufficient to result in neonatal encephalopathy almost always involves multiple organs and not just the brain (55, 56). Multisystem involvement may include acute bowel injury, renal failure, hepatic injury, cardiac damage, respiratory complications, and hematologic abnormalities (56–58).

With initial arterial hypoxemia, fetal cerebral vascular resistance can decrease by at least 50% to maintain cerebral blood flow with minimal impact on oxygen delivery (59, 60). The clinical manifestations of the redistribution of cardiac output during severe asphyxia reflect the involvement of multiple organs (eg, necrotizing enterocolitis, persistent pulmonary hypertension, hypoglycemia, disseminated intravascular coagulopathy, release of nucleated red blood cells, oliguria or anuria, hyponatremia, and fluid retention) (55, 58, 61–66).

In one study, approximately 60% of "asphyxiated" term infants exhibited single or multiple organ injury (55). In another study, severe central nervous system injury always occurred with involvement of one or more other organs (58). The presence of altered renal function (eg, oliguria) is associated with later poor neurologic outcome (58, 67).

The timing of laboratory evaluations to help assess organ injury depends on the test desired. Samples for determination of brain- and myocardial-specific creatine phosphokinase levels should be obtained as soon as possible following delivery, as the half-life of these products is measured in hours. However, cardiac troponin I may be detected up to 4 days following myocardial injury (68). Serum aminotransferase levels increase within 12 hours of ischemic injury and peak approximately 24 hours after the acute injury (69). Elevated conjugated bilirubin levels occur later and may not resolve for several weeks following hepatic injury (70). Acute elevations of

serum ammonia are associated with severe hepatic injury (71). Although an increase in urinary β_2-microglobulin is a sensitive marker of proximal tubular injury, elevated levels may not be associated with clinical renal impairment (62). Marked renal ischemia will result in acute tubular necrosis with oliguria and azotemia with progressive elevation of serum creatinine and blood urea nitrogen over several days following the acute ischemic insult (58, 67). Elevated levels of plasma concentrations of arginine vasopressin following perinatal asphyxia also are found up to 48 hours following delivery (72).

Lymphocyte and nucleated red blood cell counts are elevated among neonates with fetal asphyxial injury. Both counts appear to be more elevated and to remain elevated longer in newborns with antepartum injury than in infants with intrapartum injury. However, the rapid normalization of lymphocyte counts in the neonate limits the clinical usefulness of these counts to the first several hours after birth (64, 65).

5. Early imaging study showing evidence of acute nonfocal cerebral abnormality

Several patterns of brain injury may result from a hypoxic ischemic episode in the fetus and are dependent on the severity of cerebral hypotension, the maturity of the brain at the time of injury, and the duration of the event (44).

Early brain edema suggests recent insult. In the term infant, evaluation with MRI and diffusion imaging shows reduced motion of water within hours of the injury (47, 48). Between 24 hours and 7 days, other findings include elevated lactate levels and hyperintensity of gray matter. Later findings demonstrate cortical thinning and a decrease in the underlying white matter. In mild to moderate injury, the affected areas of the brain lie close to the inner table of the skull near the midline. In contrast, when the injury is more severe, the deeper brain substance is involved (92). Magnetic resonance imaging is optimal for the evaluation of early injury. Early detection with computed tomography and ultrasonography is of limited value, although specific findings may be observed over a period of days to weeks.

References

1. Blair E, Stanley F. When can cerebral palsy be prevented? The generation of causal hypotheses by multivariate analysis of a case-control study. Paediatr Perinat Epidemiol 1993;7:272–301. (Level II-2)

2. Blair E, Stanley FJ. Intrapartum asphyxia: a rare cause of cerebral palsy. J Pediatr 1988;112:515–9. (Level II-2)

3. Badawi N, Kurinczuk JJ, Keogh JM, Alessandri LM, O'Sullivan F, Burton PR, et al. Antepartum risk factors for newborn encephalopathy: the Western Australian case-control study. BMJ 1998;317:1549–53. (Level II-2)

4. Badawi N, Kurinczuk JJ, Keogh JM, Alessandri LM, O'Sullivan F, Burton PR, et al. Intrapartum risk factors for newborn encephalopathy: the Western Australian case-control study. BMJ 1998;317:1554–8. (Level II-2)

5. Nelson KB, Ellenberg JH. Antecedents of cerebral palsy. Univariate analysis of risk. Am J Dis Child 1985;139:1031–8. (Level II-2)

6. Nelson KB, Ellenberg JH. Antecedents of cerebral palsy. Multivariate analysis of risk. N Engl J Med 1986;315:81–6. (Level II-2)

7. Nelson KB, Leviton A. How much of neonatal encephalopathy is due to birth asphyxia? Am J Dis Child 1991;145:1325–31. (Level III)

8. Nelson KB. What proportion of cerebral palsy is related to birth asphyxia? J Pediatr 1988;112:572–4. (Level III)

9. MacLennan A. A template for defining a causal relation between acute intrapartum events and cerebral palsy: international consensus statement. BMJ 1999; 319:1054–9. (Level III)

10. Goldaber KG, Gilstrap LC 3rd, Leveno KJ, Dax JS, McIntire DD. Pathologic fetal acidemia. Obstet Gynecol 1991;78:1103–7. (Level II-3)

11. Winkler CL, Hauth JC, Tucker JM, Owen J, Bromfield CG. Neonatal complications at term as related to the degree of umbilical artery acidemia. Am J Obstet Gynecol 1991;164:637–41. (Level II-2)

12. Gilstrap LC 3rd, Leveno KJ, Burris J, Williams ML, Little BB. Diagnosis of birth asphyxia on the basis of fetal pH, Apgar score, and newborn cerebral dysfunction. Am J Obstet Gynecol 1989;161:825–30. (Level II-3)

13. Sehdev HM, Stamilio DM, Macones GA, Graham E, Morgan MA. Predictive factors for neonatal morbidity in neonates with an umbilical arterial cord pH less than 7.00. Am J Obstet Gynecol 1997;177:1030–4. (Level II-2)

14. Andres RL, Saade G, Gilstrap LC, Wilkins I, Witlin A, Zlatnik F, Hankins GV. Association between umbilical blood gas parameters and neonatal morbidity and death in neonates with pathologic fetal acidemia. Am J Obstet Gynecol 1999;181:867–71. (Level II-2)

15. Low JA, Lindsay BG, Derrick EJ. Threshold of metabolic acidosis associated with newborn complications. Am J Obstet Gynecol 1997;177:1391–4. (Level II-2)

16. Goodwin TM, Belai I, Hernandez P, Durand M, Paul RH. Asphyxial complications in the term newborn with severe umbilical acidemia. Am J Obstet Gynecol 1992;167:1506–12. (Level II-3)

17. Ruth VJ, Raivio KO. Perinatal brain damage: predictive value of metabolic acidosis and the Apgar score. BMJ 1988;297:24–7. (Level II-3)

18. Sarnat BH, Sarnat MS. Neonatal encephalopathy following fetal distress. A clinical and electroencephalographic study. Arch Neurol 1976;33:696–705. (Level III)

19. Volpe JJ. Neurology of the newborn. 4th ed. Philadelphia (PA): WB Saunders; 2001. (Level III)

20. Adamson SJ, Alessandri LM, Badawi N, Burton PR, Pemberton PJ, Stanley F. Predictors of neonatal encephalopathy in full-term infants. BMJ 1995;311: 598–602. (Level II-2)

21. Rosenbloom L. Dyskinetic cerebral palsy and birth asphyxia. Dev Med Child Neurol 1994;36:285–9. (Level III)

22. Stanley FJ, Blair E, Hockey A, Petterson B, Watson L. Spastic quadriplegia in Western Australia: a genetic epidemiological study. I: Case population and perinatal risk factors. Dev Med Child Neurol 1993;35: 191–201. (Level II-2)

23. Michaelis R, Rooschuz B, Dopfer R. Prenatal origin of congenital spastic hemiparesis. Early Hum Dev 1980;4:243–55. (Level III)

24. Nelson KB, Grether JK. Potentially asphyxiating conditions and spastic cerebral palsy in infants of normal birth weight. Am J Obstet Gynecol 1998;179:507–13. (Level II-2)

25. Govaert P, Matthys E, Zecic A, Roelens F, Oostra A, Vanzielegem B. Perinatal cortical infarction within middle cerebral artery trunks. Arch Dis Child Fetal Neonatal Ed 2000;82:F59–63. (Level III)

26. Miller V. Neonatal cerebral infarction. Semin Pediatr Neurol 2000;7:278–88. (Level III)

27. Sreenan C, Bhargava R, Robertson CM. Cerebral infarction in the term newborn: clinical presentation and long-term outcome. J Pediatr 2000;137:351–5. (Level II-2)

28. Harum KH, Hoon AH Jr, Casella JF. Factor-V Leiden: a risk factor for cerebral palsy. Dev Med Child Neurol 1999;41:781–85. (Level III)

29. Chow G, Mellor D. Neonatal cerebral ischaemia with elevated maternal and infant anticardiolipin antibodies. Dev Med Child Neurol 2000;42:412–3. (Level III)

30. Gunther G, Junker R, Strater R, Schobess K, Kurnik K, Heller C, et al. Symptomatic ischemic stroke in full-term neonates: role of acquired and genetic prothrombotic risk factors. Stroke 2000;31:2437–41. (Level II-2)

31. Kraus FT, Acheen VI. Fetal thrombotic vasculopathy in the placenta: cerebral thrombi and infarcts, coagulopathies, and cerebral palsy. Hum Pathol 1999;30: 759–69. (Level III)

32. Thorarensen O, Ryan S, Hunter J, Younkin DP. Factor V Leiden mutation: an unrecognized cause of hemiplegic cerebral palsy, neonatal stroke, and placental thrombosis. Ann Neurol 1997;42:372–5. (Level III)

33. Grether JK, Nelson KB. Maternal infection and cerebral palsy in infants of normal birth weight. JAMA 1997;278:207–11. (Level II-2)

34. Kadhim H, Tabarki B, Verellen G, De Prez C, Rona AM, Sebire G. Inflammatory cytokines in the pathogenesis of periventricular leukomalacia. Neurology 2001;56:1278–84. (Level II-2)

35. Martinez E, Figueroa R, Garry D, Visintainer P, Patel K, Verma U, et al. Elevated amniotic fluid interleukin-6 as a predictor of neonatal periventricular leukomalacia and intraventricular hemorrhage. J Matern Fetal Investig 1998;8:101–7. (Level II-2)

36. Yoon BH, Romero R, Yang SH, Jun JK, Kim IO, Choi JH, et al. Interleukin-6 concentrations in umbilical cord plasma are elevated in neonates with white matter lesions associated with periventricular leukomalacia. Am J Obstet Gynecol 1996;174:1433–40. (Level II-3)

37. Yoon BH, Jun JK, Romero R, Park KH, Gomez R, Choi JH, Kim IO. Amniotic fluid inflammatory cytokines (interleukin-6, interleukin-1 beta, and tumor necrosis factor-alpha), neonatal brain white matter lesions and cerebral palsy. Am J Obstet Gynecol 1997;177:19–26. (Level II-2)

38. Yoon BH, Romero R, Kim CJ, Koo JN, Choe G, Syn HC, et al. High expression of tumor necrosis factor-a and interleukin-6 in periventricular leukomalacia. Am J Obstet Gynecol 1997;177:406–11. (Level II-2)

39. Kraus FT. Cerebral palsy and thrombi in placental vessels of the fetus: insights from litigation. Hum Pathol 1997;28:246–8. (Level III)

40. Nelson KB, Dambrosia JM, Grether JK, Phillips TM. Neonatal cytokines and coagulation factors in children with cerebral palsy. Ann Neurol 1998;44: 665–75. (Level II-2)

41. de Veber G, Andrew M. Cerebral sinovenous thrombosis in children. N Engl J Med 2001;345:417–23. (Level II-2)

42. Barkovich AJ. MR and CT evaluation of profound neonatal and infantile asphyxia. AJNR Am J Neuroradiol 1992;13:959–72; discussion 973–5. (Level III)

43. Barkovich AJ, Westmark K, Partridge C, Sola A, Ferriero DM. Perinatal asphyxia: MR findings in the first 10 days. AJNR Am J Neuroradiol 1995;16: 427–38. (Level III)

44. Barkovich AJ. The encephalopathic neonate: choosing the proper imaging technique. AJNR Am J Neuroradiol 1997;18:1816–20. (Level III)

45. Amess PN, Penrice J, Wylezinska M, Lorek A, Townsend J, Wyatt JS, et al. Early brain proton magnetic resonance spectroscopy and neonatal neurology related to neurodevelopmental outcome at 1 year in term infants after presumed hypoxic-ischaemic brain injury. Dev Med Child Neurol 1999;41:436–45. (Level II-2)

46. Hanrahan JD, Cox IJ, Azzopardi D, Cowan FM, Sargentoni J, Bell JD, et al. Relation between proton magnetic resonance spectroscopy within 18 hours of birth asphyxia and neurodevelopment at 1 year of age. Dev Med Child Neurol 1999;41:76–82. (Level II-2)

47. Cowan FM, Pennock JM, Hanrahan JD, Manji KP, Edwards AD. Early detection of cerebral infarction and hypoxic ischemic encephalopathy in neonates using diffusion-weighted magnetic resonance imaging. Neuropediatrics 1994;25:172–5. (Level III)

48. Robertson RL, Ben-Sira L, Barnes PD, Mulkern RV, Robson CD, Maier SE, et al. MR line-scan diffusion-weighted imaging of term neonates with perinatal brain ischemia. AJNR Am J Neuroradiol 1999;20: 1658–70. (Level II-3)

49. Electronic fetal heart rate monitoring: research guidelines for interpretation. National Institute of Child Health and Human Development Research Planning Workshop. Am J Obstet Gynecol 1997;177:1385–90. (Level III)

50. Nelson KB, Dambrosia JM, Ting TY, Grether JK. Uncertain value of electronic fetal monitoring in predicting cerebral palsy. N Engl J Med 1996;334:613–8. (Level II-2)

51. Umstad MP, Permezel M, Pepperell RJ. Intrapartum cardiotography and the expert witness. Aust N Z J Obstet Gynaecol 1994;34:20–3. (Level II-3)

52. Apgar V. A proposal for a new method of evaluation of the newborn infant. Curr Res Anesth Analg 1953; 32:260–7. (Level III)

53. Apgar V, Holaday DA, James LS, Weisbrot IM, Berrien C. Evaluation of the newborn infant: second report. JAMA 1958;168:1985–8. (Level III)

54. Nelson KB, Ellenberg JH. Apgar scores as predictors of chronic neurologic disability. Pediatrics 1981;68: 36–44. (Level II-2)

55. Perlman JM, Tack ED, Martin T, Shackelford G, Amon E. Acute systemic organ injury in term infants after asphyxia. Am J Dis Child 1989;143:617–20. (Level II-2)

56. Hankins GD, Koen S, Gei AF, Lopez SM, Van Hook JW, Anderson GD. Neonatal organ system injury in acute birth asphyxia sufficient to result in neonatal encephalopathy. Obstet Gynecol 2002;99:688–91. (Level III)

57. Willis F, Summers J, Minutillo C, Hewitt I. Indices of renal tubular function in perinatal asphyxia. Arch Dis Child Fetal Neonat Ed 1997;77:F57–F60. (Level II-2)

58. Martin-Ancel A, Garcia-Alix A, Gaya F, Cabanas F, Burgueros M, Quero J. Multiple organ involvement in

perinatal asphyxia. J Pediatr 1995;127:786–93. (Level II-3)

59. Ashwal S, Dale PS, Long LD. Regional cerebral blood flow: studies in the fetal lamb during hypoxia, hypercapnia, acidosis, and hypotension. Pediatr Res 1984; 18:1309–16. (Animal study)

60. Koehler RC, Jones MD Jr, Traystman RJ. Cerebral circulatory response to carbon monoxide and hypoxic hypoxia in the lamb. Am J Physiol 1982;243: H27–H32. (Animal study)

61. Beguin F, Dunnihoo DB, Quilligan EJ. Effect of carbon dioxide elevation on renal blood flow in the fetal lamb in utero. Am J Obstet Gynecol 1974;119:630–7. (Animal study)

62. Cole JW, Portman RJ, Lim Y, Perlman JM, Robson AM. Urinary beta 2 microglobulin in full term newborns: evidence for proximal tubular dysfunction in term infants with meconium-stained amniotic fluid. Pediatrics 1985;76:958–64. (Level II-2)

63. Dauber IM, Krauss AN, Symchych PS, Auld PA. Renal failure following perinatal anoxia. J Pediatr 1976;88:851–5. (Level III)

64. Korst LM, Phelan JP, Ahn MO, Martin GI. Nucleated red blood cells: an update on the marker for fetal asphyxia. Am J Obstet Gynecol 1996;175:843–6 (Level II-2)

65. Phelan JP, Ahn MO, Korst L, Martin GI, Wang YM. Intrapartum fetal asphyxial brain injury with absent multiorgan system dysfunction. J Matern Fetal Med 1998;7:19–22. (Level III)

66. Stark H, Geiger R. Renal tubular dysfunction following vascular accidents of the kidneys in the newborn period. J Pediatr 1973;83:933–40. (Level III)

67. Perlman JM, Tack ED. Renal injury in the asphyxiated newborn infant: relationship to neurological outcome. J Pediatr 1988;113:875–9. (Level II-2)

68. Jaffe AS, Landt Y, Parvin CA, Abendschein DR, Geltman EM, Ladenson JH. Comparative sensitivity of cardiac troponin I and lactate dehydrogenase isoenzymes for diagnosing acute myocardial infarction. Clin Chem 1996;42:1770–6. (Level II-2)

69. Seeto RK, Fenn B, Rockey DC. Ischemic hepatitis: clinical presentation and pathogenesis. Am J Med 2000;109:109–13. (Level II-3)

70. Hawker F. Liver dysfunction in critical illness. Anaesth Intens Care 1991;19:165–81. (Level III)

71. Goldberg RN, Cabal LA, Sinatra FR, Plajstek CE, Hodgman JE. Hyperammonemia associated with perinatal asphyxia. Pediatrics 1979;64:336–41. (Level III)

72. Speer ME, Gorman WA, Kaplan SL, Rudolph AJ. Elevation of plasma concentrations of arginine vasopressin following perinatal asphyxia. Acta Paediatr Scand 1984;73:610–14. (Level II-2)

RESEARCH RECOMMENDATIONS

Chapter 1. Background

Neonatal Encephalopathy: Epidemiology and Long-Term Neurologic Outcomes

- Long-term follow-up studies of children enrolled in large, population-based studies should be performed to determine the full range of impairment following an unbiased assessment of neonatal encephalopathy and its subset, hypoxic–ischemic encephalopathy.

Chapter 2. Maternal Conditions

Inflammation, Infection, Coagulation Abnormalities, and Autoimmune Disorders

- Immunologic, microbiologic, and genomic studies should be performed to identify those women at greatest risk of developing intrauterine infection.

- Studies of infants born to women with thrombophilias should be conducted to determine risk for perinatal stroke and cerebral palsy and to develop clinical strategies for the prevention of disease in the neonate.

Chapter 3. Antepartum and Intrapartum Considerations and Assessment

Antepartum Events

- Reevaluate what types of focused prenatal care have the greatest potential to prevent cerebral palsy.

- Carefully define and separate antenatal clinical conditions reported to be associated with neonatal encephalopathy and cerebral palsy to ensure the relationships are valid.

Current Role of Intrapartum Electronic Fetal Heart Rate Monitoring

- Randomized prospective trials of fetal movement counting and biophysical and modified biophysical profile testing, looking at immediate and long-term outcome, are needed.

- Other forms of antenatal testing need to be investigated.

- Further characterization is needed of the physiologic mechanisms that produce hypoxic and nonhypoxic fetal heart rate change.

- Fetal heart rate change that is likely to result in hypoxic neonatal encephalopathy and cerebral palsy needs to be delineated.

- Other methods of intrapartum evaluation, such as fetal pulse oximetry and fetal electrocardiogram wave form analysis, should be evaluated further.

- Fetal heart rate patterns, if any, associated with nonhypoxic forms of neonatal encephalopathy and cerebral palsy (such as infection) should be determined.

Neonatal Neurologic Outcome Following Acute Catastrophic Intrapartum Asphyxia: The Effect of Time from Diagnosis to Delivery

- Acute catastrophic perinatal hypoxia is a rare event, and associated neonatal neurologic morbidity is uncommon. For these reasons and the host of clinical variables involved in most cases, it is impossible for a single center to collect enough cases to analyze the multiple independent factors that may affect neonatal outcome. Therefore, it would be useful to have a multi-institutional study to better evaluate the effect of acute events and long-term neonatal neurologic outcome.

Chapter 4. Fetal Considerations

Neurologic Outcome in Multiple Pregnancy

- Research is needed on preventing serious neurologic disease associated with multiple pregnancies, particularly for early delivery in multiple pregnancies with monochorionic placentation.

- Prospective studies, in which gestational age is well defined, are needed to determine if the progressive relative risk of neonatal encephalopathy after 39 weeks of gestation is preventable and if intervention could reduce or eliminate the apparent progression of risk.

Intrauterine Growth Restriction and Neonatal Encephalopathy

- Explore and elucidate the factors that control fetal growth in utero and how these factors are altered in disease states.

- Evaluate the usefulness of individual growth potential curves to identify the fetus at risk for long-term neurologic injury.

The Relative Impact of Postterm Birth Versus Postmaturity on Subsequent Neonatal Encephalopathy

- Data of this type should be confirmed by a prospective study in which gestational age is well defined to determine if the progression is preventable and if intervention could reduce or eliminate the apparent progression of risk.

Chapter 5. Neonatal Assessment

Placental Pathology Related to Neonatal Encephalopathy and Cerebral Palsy

- Further studies correlating placental pathologic findings with neonatal encephalopathy and cerebral palsy may prove useful.

Nucleated Red Blood Cells and Lymphocyte Counts and Neurologic Impairment

- Research is needed to establish the clinical utility of using nucleated red blood cell and lymphocyte levels to predict the presence of or determine the timing of neurologic insult or injury in newborns.

Chapter 6. Genetic, Anatomic, and Metabolic Etiologies of Neonatal Encephalopathy

- Research to understand the genotype and phenotype interaction may be helpful in predicting susceptibility to neonatal encephalopathy in a limited number of individuals.

Chapter 8. Criteria Required to Define an Acute Intrapartum Hypoxic Event as Sufficient to Cause Cerebral Palsy

- Basic research is needed into the initiators and mediators of neonatal encephalopathy and cerebral palsy and their long-term sequelae.

- Evaluation of other early markers of intrapartum asphyxia may be useful.

- Evaluation of the clinical utility of inflammatory mediators may be useful.

- Research focusing on the relative roles of hypoxia, infection, and other initiators of the inflammatory response is needed.

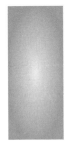

GLOSSARY

Acidemia: Increased concentration of hydrogen ions in the blood.

Pathologic acidemia: A pH level associated with adverse neurologic sequelae; the threshold for pathologic acidemia varies among research protocols, but some investigators have suggested a pH of less than 7.

Adjusted Relative Risk: The ratio of risk of disease or death among the exposed to that of the risk among the unexposed adjusted for a specific covariate (eg, maternal age, weeks of gestation, size for gestational age).

Asphyxia: A clinical situation of damaging acidemia, hypoxia, and metabolic acidosis. This definition, although traditional, is not specific to cause. A more complete definition of birth asphyxia includes a requirement for a recognizable sentinel event capable of interrupting oxygen supply to the fetus or infant. This definition fails to include conditions that are not readily recognized clinically, such as occult abruption, but is probably correct in a majority of cases.

Cerebral Palsy: Chronic static neuromuscular disability characterized by aberrant control of movement or posture, appearing early in life and not the result of recognized progressive disease.

Chorioamnionitis (clinical): A clinical presentation that may include maternal fever, maternal and fetal tachycardia, elevated white blood count, uterine tenderness, and foul-smelling vaginal effluent. The process can obviously evolve from mild subclinical to clinical disease.

Chorioamnionitis (histologic): Inflammation of the fetal membranes is a manifestation of an intrauterine infection and is frequently associated with prolonged membrane rupture and long labors. When mononuclear and polymorphonuclear leukocytes infiltrate the chorion, the resulting microscopic finding is designated chorioamnionitis.

Dysmaturity Syndrome: A dysmature fetus is characterized by wasting of subcutaneous tissue, meconium staining, peeling or desquamating skin, long fingernails, and often an alert facial expression; some are said to have "parchment-like" skin.

Hypoxemia: Decreased oxygen content in blood.

Hypoxia: Decreased level of oxygen in tissue.

Hypoxic–ischemic Encephalopathy: Also called postasphyxial encephalopathy, hypoxic–ischemic encephalopathy is a subtype of neonatal encephalopathy for which the etiology is considered to be limitation of oxygen and blood flow near the time of birth. Historically, it has been assumed that most cases of neonatal encephalopathy were hypoxic–ischemic encephalopathy, but epidemiologic studies have established that assumption is incorrect.

Intrauterine Growth Restriction: Estimated fetal weight less than the 10th percentile. The term intrauterine growth restriction includes normal fetuses at the lower end of the growth spectrum, as well as those with specific clinical conditions in which the fetus fails to achieve its inherent growth potential as a consequence of either pathologic extrinsic influences (such as maternal smoking) or intrinsic genetic defects (such as aneuploidy). Distinctions between normal and pathologic growth often cannot be made reliably in clinical practice, especially before birth. One study suggests adverse perinatal outcome generally is confined to infants with birth weights below the fifth percentile, and in most cases below the third percentile.

Ischemia: This word is derived from two Greek words: *ischein*, "to suppress," and *haima*, "blood." Thus, ischemia is the impairment of blood flow to tissues either because of constriction or frank obstruction of a blood vessel.

Near-term: Thirty-four or more completed weeks of gestation.

Negative Predictive Value: In screening and diagnostic tests, the probability that an individual with a negative test result does not have the condition is referred to as the predictive value of a negative test.

Neonatal Depression: Clinical signs of neonatal depression include low Apgar score and its components and correlates, such as hypotonia; depressed reflexes including cry, suck, Moro's embrace; decreased consciousness; difficulty in initiating and maintaining respiration; poor color; and bradycardia.

Neonatal Encephalopathy: A clinically defined syndrome of disturbed neurologic function in the earliest days of life in the term infant, manifested by difficulty with initiating and maintaining respiration, depression of tone and reflexes, subnormal level of consciousness, and often by seizures.

Nonreassuring Fetal Heart Rate Monitor Strip/Tracing: Fetal heart rate patterns that may in some cases suggest the fetus is depressed, hypoxic, or acidotic, including persistent variable decelerations of the fetal heart rate that become progressively deeper or longer lasting (generally to <70 beats per minute and lasting >60 seconds) and show persistent slow return to baseline, persistent late decelerations, prolonged deceleration (an isolated, abrupt decrease to levels below the baseline lasting at least 60–90 seconds), and sinusoidal heart rate pattern (regular oscillation of the baseline long-term variability resembling a sine wave, lasting at least 10 minutes, usually occurring at a rate of 3–5 cycles per minute and an amplitude of 5–15 beats per minute higher and lower than the baseline, not to be confused with benign small, frequent accelerations of low amplitude).

Perinatal Period: From 20 weeks of gestation to 28 days of life.

Positive Predictive Value: In screening and diagnostic tests, the probability that an individual with a positive test result is a true positive (ie, does have the condition) is referred to as the predictive value of a positive test.

Postmature-dysmature Neonate: An undernourished newborn who exhibits wasting of subcutaneous tissue, meconium staining, and peeling of skin; approximately 10–20% of true postterm fetuses exhibit these findings at birth.

Postterm Pregnancy: Gestation of 42 weeks or more (294 days or more from the first day of the last menstrual period); the term "postdates" can be simply interpreted as a pregnancy 1 or more days beyond the expected date of confinement and is *not* synonymous with postterm pregnancy.

Reassuring Fetal Heart Rate Monitor Strip/ Tracing: The absence of fetal heart rate patterns defined as nonreassuring (*see* Nonreassuring Fetal Heart Rate Monitor Strip/Tracing).

Relative Risk: The ratio of risk of disease or death among the exposed to that of the risk among the unexposed; this usage is synonymous with risk ratio. If the relative risk is higher than 1, there is a positive association between the exposure and the disease; if it is less than 1, there is a negative association.

Sensitivity: Sensitivity is the proportion of truly diseased individuals in the screened population who are identified as diseased by the screening test.

Small for Gestational Age: Infant with a birth weight at the lower extreme of the normal birth weight distribution, commonly defined as a birth weight below the 10th percentile for gestational age.

Specificity: Specificity is the proportion of truly nondiseased individuals who are so identified by the screening test.

Term Pregnancy: From 37 to 42 completed weeks of gestation since the first day of the last menstrual period

Thrombophilia: A tendency to the occurrence of thrombosis, the presence or development of an aggregation of blood factors frequently causing vascular obstruction.

INDEX

Note: Page numbers followed by letters *f* and *t* indicate figures and tables, respectively.

A

Acid-base parameters
  in humans, 31–32
  in neonatal assessment, 53
Acidemia
  definition of, 83
  pathologic, definition of, 83
Acidosis, fetal/neonatal
  as criterion for intrapartum asphyxia, 2
  intrauterine growth restriction and, 45
  metabolic, 65, as criterion for cerebral palsy, 74
  postterm pregnancy and, 47
Adjusted relative risk, definition of, 83
Age
  gestational. *See* Gestational age
  maternal, and neonatal encephalopathy, 4*t*, 25
Agency for Healthcare Research and Quality, 47
Alcohol use, and neonatal encephalopathy/cerebral palsy, 20
Amino acid metabolism disorders
  associated with neurologic manifestations, 63–65, 64*t*
  hyperammonemia with, 63–65
  neonatal hypoglycemia with, 64
Aminotransferase, serum levels, in multiorgan dysfunction, 77
Ammonia, elevated levels
  in multiorgan dysfunction, 77
  and neurologic damage, 63–65
Amnioreduction, serial, for twin-to-twin transfusion syndrome, 42
Amniotic fluid, meconium-stained, and cerebral palsy, 46–47
Amniotic fluid embolism, and neurologic outcome in fetus, 34
Anatomic abnormalities, primary, and neonatal encephalopathy, 66
Anatomic etiology, of neonatal encephalopathy, 63–69
Anesthesia, general, and neonatal encephalopathy, 6*t*

Antepartum events, and neonatal encephalopathy/cerebral palsy, 25–26
Antepartum fetal monitoring
  and neonatal encephalopathy, 27
  predictive value of, 27
Antiepileptic drugs, 19
Antiphospholipid antibody, 18
Antithrombin III deficiency, 18, 75
Apgar score, 54–55
  and cerebral palsy, 6–7, 55, 55*t*, 76–77
  in encephalopathy evaluation, 54–55
  factors affecting, 54
  5-minute
    normal, 54
    relative risk of death and disabilities according to, 54–55, 55*t*
  infection and, 14–15
  and intrapartum asphyxia, 2, 54–55
  intrapartum fetal monitoring and, 27
  and long-term neurologic outcome, 2, 6–7, 54–55
  "Use and Abuse of the Apgar Score" (ACOG), 54
  "Use and Misuse of the Apgar Score" (ACOG), 54
Apoptosis, and neonatal encephalopathy, 17
Arginine vasopressin, 59
Argininosuccinic acid deficiency, 64, 64*t*
Aspartate, metabolic disorders and, 65
Asphyxia, definition of, 83
Astrocytic swelling, hyperammonemia and, 65
Asymmetric intrauterine growth restriction, 43–44
Attention disorders, intrauterine growth restriction and, 45
Attributable fraction, 7
Auscultatory fetal heart rate monitoring, 27
Autoimmune disorders, and neonatal encephalopathy/cerebral palsy, 19

B

Bacterial vaginosis
  and chorioamnionitis, 17
  and preterm birth, 15–16

Basal ganglia injury
  intrapartum asphyxia and, 8–9, 29
  neuroimaging of, 56–57
Beneficial Aspects of Antenatal Magnesium (BEAM) Trial, 71–72
Betamethasone
  for prevention of intraventricular hemorrhage, 71
  for prevention of periventricular leukomalacia, 71
Bilirubin, serum levels, in multiorgan dysfunction, 77
Biophysical profile testing, and neurologic outcome, 27
Birth asphyxia, 2. *See also* Intrapartum asphyxia
  definition of, 83
  International Classification of Diseases-9 criteria for, 54
  incidence of, 3
Birth order, and neurologic outcome in multiple pregnancy, 40
Birth weight
  and cerebral palsy, 1
  infection/inflammation and, 15–16
  in multiple pregnancy, and neurologic outcome, 39–40
  and neonatal encephalopathy, 1, 5*t*, 43
  in postterm pregnancy, 47
Bleeding, in pregnancy, and neonatal encephalopathy/cerebral palsy, 4–5, 5*t*, 13–14, 26
Blood flow
  cerebral, neuroimaging of, 55
  responses to intrapartum asphyxia, 8
Blood gas analysis, 31–32, 53
Body length, neonatal, and intrauterine growth restriction, 43–44
Brachial plexus injury, postterm pregnancy and, 47
Bradycardia, in cerebral palsy, 76
Brain damage. *See* Neonatal encephalopathy
Branched-chain amino acid disorders, 63

C

California Child Health and Development Study, 25–26
Capacitance effect, in twin pregnancy, 42